THREAD LIFTING

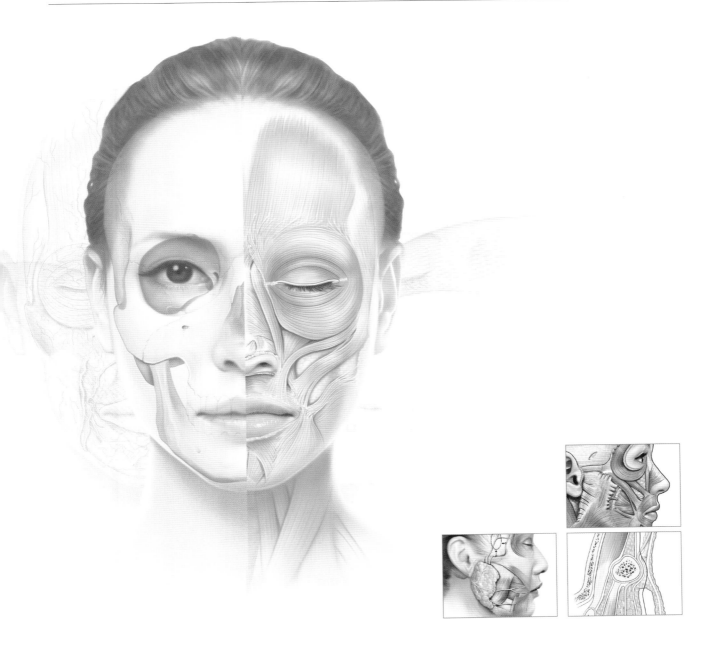

KOONJA

Textbook of Absorbable Thread Lifting

First edition printed | August 31, 2018
First edition published | September 14, 2018

Written by	Seung-hoon Kang, Bong-il Rho, Seong-jae Youn
Published by	Ju-yeon Jang
Planned by	Sung-jae Lee
Editing Design by	Eun-jung Yang
Cover Design by	Jae-wook Kim
Illustrations by	Ho-hyeon Lee
Produced by	Sang-hyeon Shin
Publishing House	Koonja Publishing, Inc.
	Registration No. 4-139 (June 24, 1991)
	Paju Publishing Complex, 338, Hoedong-gil (474-1 Seopae-dong),
	Paju-si, Gyeonggi-do, South Korea (10881)
	Telephone : (031) 943-1888 Fax : (031) 955-9545
	Website : www.koonja.co.kr

ISBN 979-11-5955-356-1
Price $180

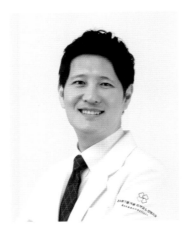

Seung-hoon Kang

- Chief, 4 Seasons Dermatology Clinic
- Board of Dermatology
- Graduated from Inje University School of Medicine
- Director of Academic Affairs, Korean Association of Anti-aging Medicine
- Director of Academic Affairs, Association of Korean Corrective Dermatology
- Director of Publishing, Association of Korean Dermatology

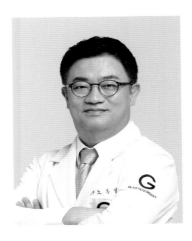

Bong-il Rho

- Chief, Glovi Plastic Surgery Clinic
- Board of plastic surgery
- Graduated from Soonchunhyang University School of Medicine
- Former Planning Director of the Board of Minimally Invasive Plastic Surgery Research, Korean Society of Plastic and Reconstructive Surgeons
- Former Standing Director, Korean Association of Clinical Plastic Surgeons
- Former Chairman of the Board of Minimally Invasive Plastic Surgery Research, Korean Society of Plastic and Reconstructive Surgeons

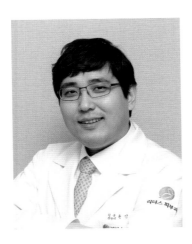

Seong-jae Youn

- Chief, Leaders Clinic Apgujeong
- Board of Dermatology
- Graduated from Seoul National University School of Medicine
- Director of Education, Research Board of the Korea Association of Anti-aging Medicine
- Adjunct Associate Professor, Sungkyunkwan University School of Medicine

Beginning with the Aptos lift in the late 1980s, thread lifting has seen continual advances and improvement during the last 40 years. Nevertheless, for much of its long history, thread lifting was not a widely known procedure among physicians or the general public. This changed 10 years ago with the development of absorbable thread lifting techniques using polydioxanone (PDO), which precipitated the popularization of a new concept of lifting to achieve not only elevation but also tissue stimulation and regeneration and began a new chapter in the history of thread lifting.

We have accumulated much experience with both absorbable and nonabsorbable thread lifting and learned a lot about their differences and respective strengths and weaknesses. However, there have still not been many studies or research papers on the theoretical background and practical techniques for absorbable thread lifting. While foreign physicians have shown great interest in absorbable thread lifting during overseas presentations and meetings in Korea, we have also felt that these physicians often gain doubts about the nature of the procedure, since they have not seen related textbooks.

We wrote this book to be a cornerstone of absorbable thread lifting, which has the potential to develop as an area of academic interest both in Korea and worldwide. Although writing this book took more time and effort than expected, in retrospect, there is still much room for improvement. We have also experienced a great amount of change and improvement in these 2 years, but we consider this a beginning and plan to further supplement and enhance this content in the future.

This book aims to describe a general, objective technique that can be used by anyone to produce similar results, rather than the individual experiences and techniques of the authors. Depending on the surgeon's skill, it is also possible to use only monofilament thread, and in the future, as we gain more experience, we will include an explanation of a method that also uses cog thread at a level that is suited to novices and experts alike. Above all, we aimed to discuss various real clinical cases, in order to help readers familiarize the technique in practice.

We want to express our gratitude to Koonja Publishing Company's CEO Ju-Yeon Jang, Section Manager Ho-Hyun Lee, and Assistant Manager Eun-Hee Jo who provided material and moral assistance for the publication of this book. We would also like to thank all the esteemed teachers and colleagues who have helped us to work diligently at our respective hospitals. We hope that this book will contribute in some way to the academic advancement of absorbable thread lifting.

Seung-Hoon Kang, Bong-Il Rho, Seong-Jae Youn

"From the foundations to learning···
A new textbook and standard for thread lifting"

Ee Seok Lim

It has been over 10 years since thread lifting was first introduced in Korea. During that time, a number of texts on thread lifting have been published, but there has not yet been a book discussing every aspect of thread lifting in detail, from A to Z.

This book not only contains basic information about thread-based procedures but also includes various methods and the full sum of practical knowledge that has been acquired over the years. For this reason, I consider this book an introduction for physicians hoping to begin thread lifting and a bible of thread lifting to answer the unresolved questions of physicians already practicing the technique.

I have known the authors for a long time, and they have a wealth of experience with thread lifting and broad medical knowledge, based on which they vividly explain thread lifting not as a singular method of wrinkle correction but in terms of its diverse applications in different areas. Moreover, the three authors present a new paradigm for absorbable thread lifting by combining their individual opinions and methods.

Unlike previous textbooks, the use of actual case studies and experiences involves the readers and keeps them fascinated. I was especially impressed by the extensiveness of information on thread lifting, including authors' research results, actual histological findings, and clinical experiences.

In particular, diversification and popularization of a technique inevitably leads to an increase in adverse effects. This book discusses truly important issues in depth, such as areas of caution in reducing adverse effects and methods of coping with any adverse effects that should arise. Thus, I have no doubt that this book, which contains everything you want to know about thread lifting, including the latest clinical trial results, various techniques, and prevention of and response to adverse effects, will become readers' best and most reliable guidebook.

Chief, Lim Ee Seok Theme Dermatological Clinic
Chair, Korean Association of Corrective Dermatology
Chair, Korean Society of Hair Restoration Treatment
Former Chair, Association of Korean Dermatologists
Former Auditor, Korean Society of Dermatologic Laser Surgery

Contents

Contents

TEXTBOOK OF ABSORBABLE THREAD LIFTING

Chapter 01

The History and Theoretical Background of Thread Lifting

SECTION 1   History and Theoretical Background

SECTION 1

History and Theoretical Background

Various surgical methods, peeling, and laser/radiofrequency therapy have been used for correction of wrinkles or stretched skin, and these methods are still being improved. In particular, technologically advanced products using laser, radiofrequency, or ultrasound-based methods are being released with rapid turnover.

Although surgery is effective, it can lead to adverse effects, such as hematoma, neurological injury, and scarring, and the long recovery time, with significantly delayed return to social activities. Moreover, surgical approaches are less accessible owing to the relatively high level of skill required. Wrinkle correction methods using laser, radiofrequency, or ultrasound therapy are technically easy with few side effects. However, although the recovery period is short and patients soon return to social activities, these methods require expensive equipment and the treatment effect is lower than that of surgery.

In contrast, thread lifting is often used for wrinkle correction because of its low initial cost, rapid return to social activities, high patient satisfaction, and minimal adverse effects.

Non-absorbable thread lifting has a long history, but was seldom used because of a debate regarding its effect and persistence (transcutaneous face lift). In 2002, Dr. Gordon Sasaki published a thread lifting method using Gore-Tex in Plastic and Reconstructive Surgery; although the thread was commercially available in Korea, several issues limited the use of this method. Thus, thread lifting methods using an unmodified, plain suture have been used for a long time but only infrequently.

Thread lifting began to gain popularity in Korea with the development of methods using barbed/cog threads.

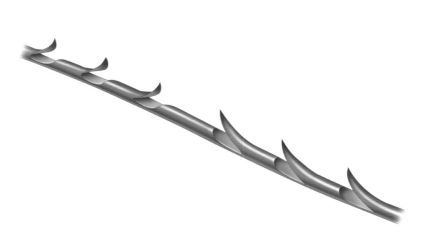

Figure 1-1. APTOS Lift®

Developed by Dr. Ruff in the early 1990s, barbed thread lifting achieved global recognition and popularity following improvements by Dr. Sulamanidze in the late 1990s, global patenting was obtained in 1999, and a paper was published in 2001 (Figure. 1–1). Suturing using a unidirectional barbed thread was reported by Al Camo in 1964. Suturing using a bidirectional barbed thread was reported by Alan McKenzie in 1967.

The lifting method using approximately 10 cm of non-absorbable bidirectional barbed thread is called the Aptos (standing for antiptosis) lift.

In 2004, contour threads (Featherlift Extended Aptos Length Threads) were approved by the US Food and Drug Administration (FDA) for use in face lifting and suturing, but they cannot be used in Korea since they were not approved by the Korea Food and Drug Administration (KFDA).

In 2003, barbed thread lifting became popular in Korea for the first time with the introduction of the Aptos lift, but because Asians typically have thicker and heavier skin than Westerners, the lifting effect is inevitably reduced. Moreover, Asians have more developed cheekbones, and the bidirectional barbs used in reducing the prominence of the nasolabial folds have the drawback of making the cheekbones appear even larger.

This led to the interest in methods where sutures are placed in a firm tissue and the sagging tissue is lifted as a whole. In 2004, the "suture suspension for lifting method," developed by Bulgaria's Dr. Serdev using elastic thread and specialized instruments, was introduced in Korea, but the thread used by Dr. Serdev was not granted domestic approval, and the method was not commonly used due to the lack of effect persistence.

Later, several threads were developed for fixed methods, but the effects were disappointing, and these threads were rarely used. This is because of the so-called "cheese-wiring effect," in which movement of the muscles of facial expression and the downward pull of gravity on the tissue cause the thread, which is made into a loop and used to create upward tension, to cut into the tissue. This, in turn, reduces the strength with which the thread can hold the tissue. In order to overcome these limitations, methods were devised using thread with the addition of

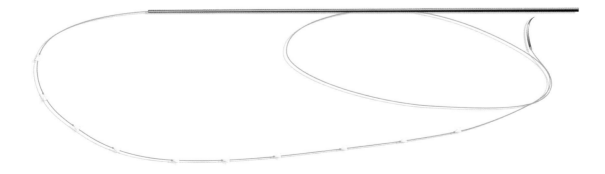

Figure 1–2. Silhouette lift®

barbs in the loop to lift the sagging tissue as a whole.

In 2007, the Silhouette lift became available in Korea, lifting tissue with a non-absorbable suture thread that has cones, rather than barbs. Although this treatment was highly effective and relatively persistent, it did not become popular because of the difficulty of the technique, requiring an incision in the scalp, and the relatively high cost of materials (Figure 1-2).

A lifting method using a long, barbed, non-absorbable suture thread without the need for scalp incision was first used in Korea in 2007, immediately after product approval. However, this method also failed to become popular since it requires large quantities of thread to be inserted, the thread cannot be absorbed, and the procedure is technically difficult, requiring fixation in the deep temporal fascia.

While there had previously been a trend for non-absorbable thread, from the 2010s, absorbable thread lifting techniques began to gain attention. In particular, in Korea, there was a massive growth in techniques attaching non-barbed polydioxanone (PDO) thread to a needle and placing it in the subcutaneous layer. Methods using PDO thread have relatively low cost of materials, short procedure time, and rapid recovery time. In contrast, its effect is relatively lesser compared with those of fixed methods, and the persistence time is short. To improve these shortcomings, from around 2012, thread lifting was performed using floating type methods with 10-15 cm of barbed absorbable thread.

Later, lifting would also be performed with fixed methods using at least 40 cm of barbed thread. Among the authors of this book, Bong-Il Rho (Glovi Plastic Surgery Clinic) presented his experiences of fixed thread lifting using long barbed absorbable thread consisting of a copolymer of glycolic acid and trimethylene carbonate to the Chinese Annual Meeting of Minimally Invasive Aesthetic Medicine in September 2013. Subsequently, various types of absorbable threads have been developed and commercialized.

Barbed thread has been manufactured since 2013, with the barbs made by molding the thread rather than the conventional method of cutting with a knife.

Lately, barbed thread is even being made by pressing into metal molds under gentle heating. Since this thread contains more barbs than previous types of molded thread, it is thought to pull more tightly on the tissue.

Judging by the history of advances in suture thread, the effectiveness of thread lifting is limited by its persistence. Absorbable thread is thought to be ideal for thread lifting, since it is possible to perform multiple procedures until the age when a facelift is required. Meanwhile, in order to increase the lifting effect on sagging tissue, it is thought to be beneficial to use a molded thread with numerous strong barbs, made from a material that is absorbed slowly.

[References]

1. Meloplication of the Malar Fat Pads by Percutaneous Cable-Suture Technique for Midface Rejuvenation: Outcome Study(392 Cases, 6 Years' Experience. Plastic & Reconstructive Surgery. 09/2002: 110(2):635-54

2. Technique and uses for absorbable barbed sutures. Aethet Surg 2006:26:620-628

3. Suture suspensions for lifting or volume augmentation in face and body, presented at the 2nd annual meeting of the national Bulgarian society for aethetic surgery and awthetic medicine, Sofia, 18, March 1994, Int J Aesth Cosm, 2001,1:1, 2561-2568

4. Facial lifting with APTOS threads. Int J Cosmetic Surg Aethetic Dermatolo 2001:4:275-281

5. "Waptos lift"-Dr. Woffles, Nonsurgical face lifting with long barbed suture slings: The Woffles lift. Journal fur Aesthetische Chirurgie 1.2013.6:13-20

TEXTBOOK OF ABSORBABLE
THREAD LIFTING

Chapter 02

Anatomical Background of Thread Lifting

SECTION 1

Layers of the Face

The face consists of numerous layers, from the skin to the bone. In the most common classification used by Mendelson et al., the face is divided into 5 layers. Starting from the surface and moving deeper, the face consists of the skin, superficial fat, muscle layer (including the superficial musculoaponeurotic system [SMAS]), deep fat, and bone. However, some of the facial muscles are located superficial to the SMAS, while some are located deeper. Moreover, the muscles each have different trajectories, originating from the bone and sometimes inserting into the skin, meaning that the 5 layer classification above is not always applicable.

In thread lifting, the most important structure is the fascia. The fascia of the face can be divided into the superficial and deep fasciae.

The superficial fascia is the SMAS, which is thicker toward the parotid gland and gradually becomes thinner moving in the anterior direction. The SMAS is connected to the platysma muscle inferiorly and the superficial temporal fascia superiorly.

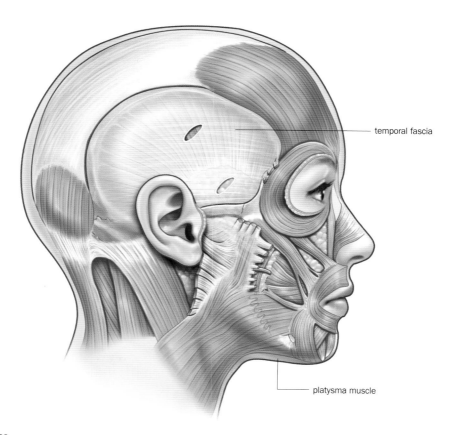

temporal fascia

platysma muscle

Figure 2–1. Facial muscles

The deep fascia of the face is called the masseteric fascia when it covers the masseter muscle and the parotid fascia or parotic capsule when it surrounds the parotid gland. In conjunction, it is called the parotid masseteric or parotidomasseteric fascia. This deep fascia connects at the neck with the deep cervical fascia, which covers the sternocleidomastoid (SCM), and connects superiorly with the deep temporal fascia, which covers the temporalis muscle.

Thus, the superficial and deep fasciae of the face are partially connected, mostly in areas with retaining ligaments. During thread lifting, the thread is passed through some areas where the superficial and deep fasciae are tightly attached, such as below the parotid gland or zygoma and the anterior margin of the masseter muscle. As a result, the surgeon will feel some resistance when placing a trocar or large needle in these areas for thread lifting.

In addition, the superficial fascia forms a firm connection with the deep fascia as it passes inferiorly along the posterior margin of the platysma muscle, lateral to the parotid gland. This area has been given different names by different researchers (Figure 2-1); Fumas and Mendelson described this as the platysma auricular ligament, while Stuzin identified it as the parotid cutaneous ligament. Regardless of nomenclature, this area is clinically important since it provides a fixation point for the soft tissue below the ear using a short, barbed thread.

In cog thread lifting, the fascia is important in maintaining support as an attachment point for the thread. In the temporal area, we use a long thread fixed to the deep temporal fascia, and in the midface, we use a normal thread fixed to the superficial fascia.

SECTION 2

Vasculature and Nerves

The important vascular, neural, and glandular structures of the face are located between the fat and retaining ligaments. Although thread lifting does not cause the same severe complications or skin necrosis as filler procedure, if the thread is placed near the surface, it can lead to an uneven appearance or visible thread postoperatively. If the thread penetrates the parotid gland, it can result in sequelae such as salivary leakage. Therefore, it is essential to have an understanding of the basic anatomy.

During filler procedures, it is important for the surgeon to be familiar with the locations of the facial, supraorbital, supratrochlear, and superficial temporal arteries to avoid injecting the filler into the vasculature. Knowing the locations of blood vessels is useful in thread lifting to minimize swelling and bruising due to minor bleeding.

The superficial temporal artery, which is an important consideration when fixing cog thread to the temporal area, is usually known to pass superolaterally through the lateral edge of the eyebrow. However, there is a significant interindividual variation that makes it difficult to

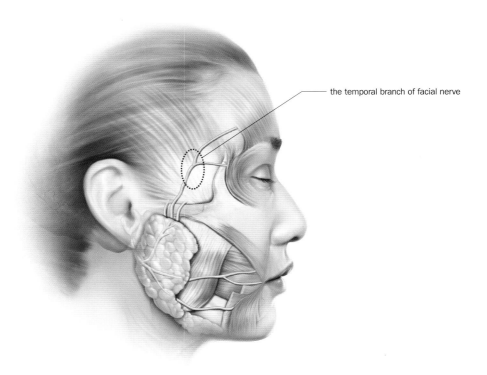

the temporal branch of facial nerve

Figure 2-2. Temporal branch of the facial nerve

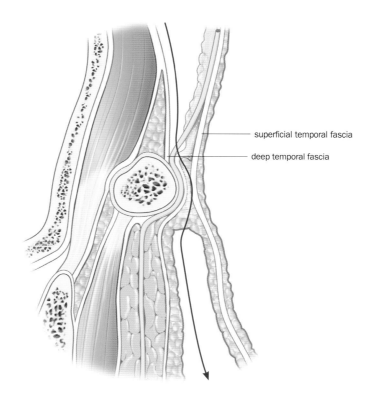

superficial temporal fascia

deep temporal fascia

Figure 2-3. Ideal path of thread (arrow)

confirm the trajectory of the superficial temporal artery based only on its relationships with surrounding structures.

Because the superficial temporal artery is wide, its pulse can sometimes be palpated. Therefore, we advise to feel for a pulse at the planned fixation point when using cog-type anchor thread to check for the passage of the artery. The superficial temporal artery is mostly surrounded by the SMAS, traveling superomedially past the lateral edge of the eyebrow and gradually becoming closer to the surface, traveling superficial to the frontalis muscle as it approaches the midline of the face. In approximately 50% of cases, the superficial temporal artery forms an arcade anastomosing the supraorbital and supratrochlear arteries.

When using the cog-less PDO thread or short-cog thread, nerve injury is not a concern because the thread is mainly placed on the subcutaneous fat layer. As discussed above, most of the nerves of the face are found deeper than the deep fascia.

One area that does require caution is fixation of long cog thread in the temporal area. Although the fixation point differs among surgeons, when the thread is fixed to the deep temporal fascia, the trocar or cannula may pass between the superficial and deep fasciae at the location of the temporal branch of the facial nerve (Figures 2-2, 2-3). In this case, it is natural to be concerned about facial nerve injury caused by the trocar or cannula, but this does not occur as readily as might be imagined.

This is because, first, if the surgeon proceeds slowly and gently, it is generally possible to avoid the nerve with the tip of the cannula or trocar and, second, the temporal branch of the facial nerve divides into multiple strands toward its distal end, and so one or two strands may be injured without causing any major clinical problems.

Indeed, while there have been some case reports of injury to this nerve during facelift surgery, there are currently no case reports of injury while inserting the trocar or cannula for thread lifting. Therefore, there is no need for undue concern about nerve injury during noninvasive thread lifting.

TEXTBOOK OF ABSORBABLE THREAD LIFTING

Chapter 03

Classification and Types of Thread

SECTION 1

Classification of Threads by Material

Generally, the suture thread is divided into absorbable and non-absorbable thread, depending on whether it is absorbed by the body. It can also be classified into natural and synthetic thread by material or monofilament and multifilament thread by the number of filaments it contains.

In this section, we summarize the characteristics of several absorbable threads relative to polydioxanone (PDO), which is currently the most commonly used type of absorbable thread.

1. Catgut

This is a natural (non-synthetic) absorbable thread isolated from pure connective tissue (usually collagen). However, it is not used lately due to poor tensile strength and knot stability and because it causes a strong tissue response.

2. Polyglycolic acid (PGA)

This was the first synthetic absorbable thread and can be manufactured in monofilament or braided forms. The tensile strength decreases to 89% after 7 days in the body, 63% after 14 days, and 17% after 21 days. The thread is absorbed by a process of hydrolysis, and complete absorption takes 90-120 days. The tensile strength is relatively good, and the knot stability is excellent.

3. Polyglactic acid

This thread is made from a copolymer of lactide and glycolide, coated with a synthetic lubricant and made into a braided form. The tensile strength decreases to 65% after 2 weeks and 40% after 3 weeks. The thread is absorbed by hydrolysis, and complete absorption takes 60-90 days.

4. PDO

This is a synthetic monofilament thread. Chemically, it is a polymer of infinitely repeated ether-ester units (Figure 3-1).

The thread is absorbed by hydrolysis, and the final product is excreted in the urine or in the breath in the form of CO_2. The tensile strength decreases to 74% after 2 weeks in the body, 50% after 4 weeks, and 25% after 6 weeks. Complete absorption occurs within 180 days. Since it is a monofilament, it does not cause much of an inflammatory response and is currently the

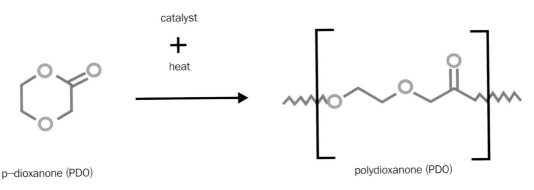

catalyst
+
heat

p–dioxanone (PDO)

polydioxanone (PDO)

Figure 3–1. The chemical structural equation of polydioxanone

most commonly used absorbable thread for thread lifting because it is highly cost effective. Given that the thread is absorbed by hydrolysis, it rapidly breaks down in moist environments. Therefore, it is best to use the thread immediately from its sealed packaging. In the case that leftover thread needs to be stored, it should be kept in an environment with minimal moisture.

5. Polytrimethylene carbonate

This is a synthetic monofilament thread made of a copolymer of glycolide and trimethylene carbonate. Like PDO, the thread has excellent tensile strength and causes less tissue response. In addition, the thread is approximately 60% more flexible than PDO, making it easy to manipulate during surgery.

The tensile strength decreases to 81% after 14 days, 59% after 28 days, and 30% after 42 days. The thread is absorbed by hydrolysis, and complete absorption takes 180-210 days. The drawback of this thread is that it is more expensive than other absorbable threads.

SECTION 2

Classification of Threads by Shape

Here, we classify absorbable threads by their shape. As in the Table 5–1, we classified threads based on the presence or absence of barbs; structural modifications, such as twisting or combining multiple strands; and material modifications.

First, threads can be divided into those with a smooth surface, without any particular surface modifications, and those with an uneven surface due to the addition of barbs or other three-dimensional structures.

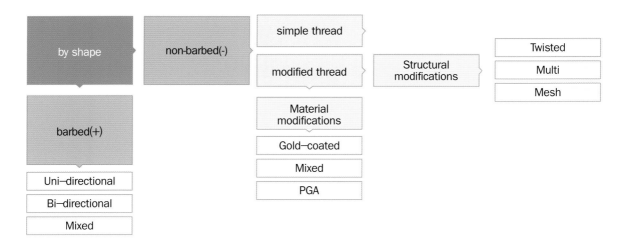

Figure 3-2. Classification of thread by shape

Non-barbed thread can be further subdivided into simple threads that are preloaded into a needle and threads with various structural or material modifications (Figure 3-2).

2-1. Non-barbed threads

1. Simple, plain, mono-PDO thread (Figure 3-5)

This is thread that has been cut to a certain length before loading into a needle, folding the thread back at the tip of the needle and fixing the thread with a sponge or similar material. The needle width, needle length, and thread length are displayed on the product, and the appropriate thread can be selected according to its intended purpose.

It is most common to use a single strand of thread, but multi-strand sutures are sometimes used with two or more threads loaded in the same needle.

2. Structurally/materially modified thread

1) Structurally modified non-barbed thread

(1) Twisted (Figure 3-3)

After inserting simple, non-barbed thread into the needle, the thread is coiled around the needle. Due to its appearance, this thread is also sometimes called cyclone/tornado/hurricane thread.

(2) Multi (Figure 3-6)

Multiple strands of thread are inserted into the same needle. This thread is available in both

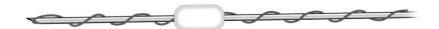

Figure 3-3. Twisted

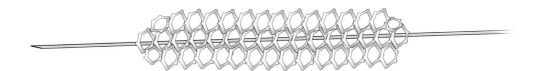

Figure 3-4. Mesh

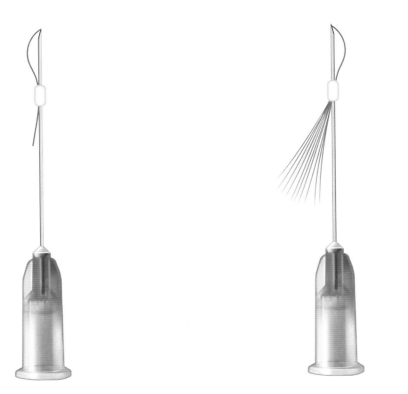

Figure 3-5. Simple, non-barbed thread   Figure 3-6. Multifilament thread

simple and twisted forms. Some products are made by braiding two or three strands of modified thread into a single thread before insertion into the needle.

(3) Mesh (Figure 3-4)

This is a PDO thread that has been made into a mesh shape. Since the area in contact with the skin is broader, it is beneficial for skin rejuvenation.

2) Materially modified non-barbed thread

(1) Gold-coated thread

This is a PDO thread that has been coated with absorbable gold using nano-coating technology. According to a paper published by Masakazu et al., albeit using non-absorbable thread, gold-coated thread resulted in greater collagen production in 7 months than barbed thread.

Gold-coated thread can be expected to be more effective than plain PDO thread in producing a clear complexion and eliminating micro-wrinkles via collagen production. However, it can lead to adverse reactions such as pigmentation caused by hypersensitivity reaction when laser toning is performed using a 1064-nm Q-switched Nd-YAG laser with gold-coated thread placed on the surface layer. For this reason, it is important to check whether gold-coated thread has been placed prior to any toning treatment and proceed with caution.

(2) PDO/PGA mixed thread

This is a thread prepared by braiding PDO and PGA threads into a single strand and inserting it into a needle. The intention is to induce more collagen synthesis, since PGA has a greater propensity to induce an inflammatory response. The surgeon needs to be aware that the thread manufactured in this way can cause a more severe inflammatory response than monofilament thread. We believe that further clinical trials and experience are required to properly evaluate this thread.

2-2. Barbed threads

1. By barb direction

1) Unidirectional barbed thread (Figure 3-7)

The first method of making barbed thread is to have all the barbs facing the same direction. Prepared by inserting some of the thread into a needle, folding at the needle tip, and fixing the rest of the thread outside the needle, the unidirectional barbed thread was used initially. However, a single operation did not provide effective lifting owing to insufficient fixation, so recently the bidirectional or multidirectional barbed thread has been more commonly used.

Another method is to use a needle to pierce the skin, insert two unidirectional barbed threads at a slight angle, tie the threads at the entrance, and push the knot under the skin.

2) Bidirectional barbed thread (Figure 3-8)

The bidirectional barbed thread is made with barbs projecting in opposite directions. This is currently the most commonly used type of barbed thread for absorbable thread lifting procedures. The barbs project in opposite directions on either side of a central point. In thread lifting, it is common to use a thread with the barbs projecting toward each other, but sometimes a thread with the barbs projecting away from each other is used.

3) Multidirectional/mixed barbed thread (Figure 3-9)

This thread includes those with several repeating sections of bidirectional barbs and those with every other barb facing the opposite direction. Compared to the bidirectional barbed thread, the multidirectional barbed thread reduces the change of migration, and this characteristic is often used alone or in combination with the bidirectional thread.

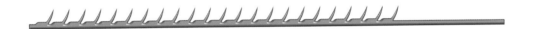

Figure 3-7. Unidirectional barbed thread

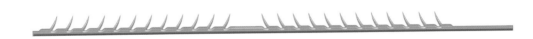

Figure 3-8. Bidirectional barbed thread

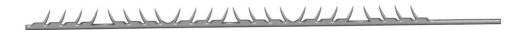

Figure 3-9. Multidirectional/mixed barbed thread

2. By method of barb fabrication

1) Cutting type (Figure 3–10)

The first method of making barbed thread is to make fine cuts on the surface of the thread. The advantage of this method is that it is easy to make the barbs; however, since the surface of the thread is cut, tensile strength decreases slightly compared to the unmodified thread.

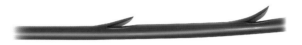

Figure 3–10. Cutting–type thread

Barb geometry

Gregory Ruff reported that barb shape affected the holding and tensile strengths of the thread. In his study, Ruff found that making deeper barbs resulted in decreased tensile strength in the thread as a whole and arranging the barbs in a spiral pattern, rather than in a straight line, helped the thread to hold the skin.

In another study, Jeffrey Zeruby et al. reported that holding strength was improved and barbs were less susceptible to bending when the number of barbs was greater and the barbs were wider, thicker, and vertically arranged.

2) Molding type (Figure 3–11)

The drawback of the cutting-type barbed thread is reduced tensile strength compared to that of the uncut thread. To eliminate this problem, there have recently been barbed threads produced without cutting, by using a specially shaped metal mold and applying high pressure to parts of the thread other than the barbs. This process is sometimes accompanied by heating, but since high temperatures can reduce the thread's tensile strength, when selecting a product, it is important to consider that threads that have undergone minimal heating have the best tensile strength.

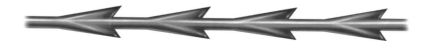

Figure 3–11. Molding–type thread

[References]

1. Kurita M, Matsumoto D, Kato H, Araki J, Higashino T, Fujino T, Takasu K, Yoshimura K. Tissue reactions to cog structure and pure gold in lifting threads: a histological study in rats. Aesthet Surg J. 2011 Mar;31(3):347-51.

2. Ruff G., Technique and uses for absorbable barbed sutures. Aesthet Surg J. 2006 Sep-Oct;26(5):620-8.

3. Zaruby J, Gingras K, Taylor J, Maul D., An in vivo comparison of barbed suture devices and conventional monofilament sutures for cosmetic skin closure: biomechanical wound strength and histology. Aesthet Surg J. 2011 Feb;31(2):232-40.

TEXTBOOK OF ABSORBABLE THREAD LIFTING

Chapter **04**

Preoperative Preparations

SECTION 1

Consultation

The most important aspects of consultation with patients who want thread lifting are to understand the extent of the patient's expectations and predict the actual outcomes of the procedure.

If the patient's expectations are too high, they may be disappointed even if the outcome is good. This is because thread lifting is not yet widespread, and patients are unfamiliar with the procedure and extent of improvement. During consultation, it is important for the physician to lift the patient's face manually, to both simulate the outcome of the procedure in advance and identify the trajectory of the ideal lifting line.

In summary, the surgeon should ascertain the patient's expectations through a meticulous consultation and make efforts to align these expectations with the realistic predicted outcomes of the procedure. To this end, discriminating clinical indications should be prioritized. Referring to the table of positive and negative factors below will help in predicting outcomes and consulting with patients (Table 4-1).

Table 4-1. Prognostic factors for thread lifting

Favorable prognostic factors	Unfavorable prognostic factors
Unfavorable prognostic factors	Old age (50 – 69 years)
Relatively thin skin	Relatively thick skin
Less prominent cheekbones	More prominent cheekbones
Flatter cheeks	Fuller cheeks
Narrower jaw	Square jaw
More concerned about the jawline (hoping to make a "V–line" jaw)	More concerned about correcting perioral wrinkles/marionette lines

SECTION 2

Imaging

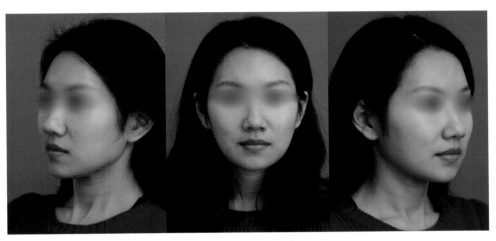

Figure 4-1. Sample preoperative photographs (frontal, left, and right 45° oblique)

Clinical photographs should be taken in the frontal and left and right 45° oblique views and stored for comparison with postoperative photographs. Take care to maintain the same lighting and angles for pre- and postoperative photographs (Figure 4-1).

SECTION 3

Surgical Preparation

1. Surgical position

The standard position for the procedure is the supine position, with the patient lying flat on their back. However, we actually recommend operating with the patient in an extended neck Trendelenburg position, with the body tilted slightly posteriorly and the neck placed in extension (Figure 4-2). In this position, gravity causes the targeted tissues to naturally shift in the intended lift direction. This provides gentle fixation that can help achieve favorable results.

This position can also reduce adverse outcomes that may occur in the standard position, such as excessive traction, or an unnatural face shape or facial expressions postoperatively, with the face appearing to expand laterally.

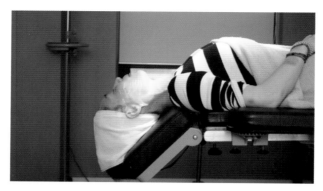

Figure 4-2. Patient position for thread lifting (extended neck Trendelenburg position)

2. Instruments

For monofilament thread lifting, it is possible to perform the procedure without any specialized equipment, as long as an antiseptic agent and drapes are available. However, when using barbed thread, instruments are required to place the thread and then remove the remaining thread from the skin.

The instruments we use with the barbed thread are listed below (Figure 4-3).

1) Awl (Figure 4-4)

This instrument is used to penetrate the skin. Although an 18-G or 21-G needle can be used, using an awl can reduce the risk of bruising due to vascular rupture.

2) Anesthetic cannula (Figure 4-5)

This instrument is used to inject tumescent anesthesia prior to thread lifting. The risk of bruising is reduced compared to anesthesia induction using a standard needle. In our experience using a cannula or needle larger than 21 G can cause severe pain, so it is preferable to use a smaller needle if possible.

3) Temporal needle/hook (Figure 4-6)

The temporal fascia is a very robust tissue below the scalp. When using an anchoring thread, the temporal needle/hook is used to fix the thread to the temporal fascia.

4) Cannula/stylet (Figures 4-7, 4-8)

The above instruments are used to place the thread inside the skin. In thread lifting, a cannula containing a blunt stylet is placed at the site of thread insertion. After removing the

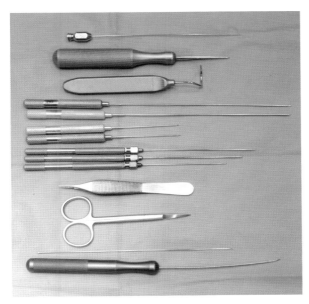

Figure 4-3. Instruments used in thread lifting

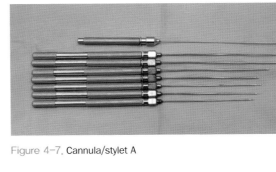

Figure 4-7. Cannula/stylet A

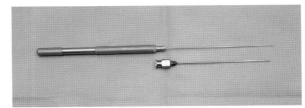

Figure 4-8. Cannula/stylet B

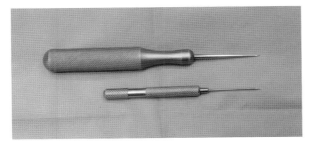

Figure 4-4. Awl

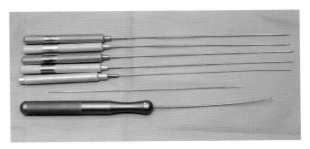

Figure 4-9. Cannula/stylet A

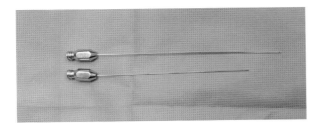

Figure 4-5. Anesthesia cannula

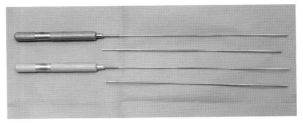

Figure 4-10. Cannula/stylet B

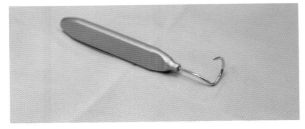

Figure 4-6. Temporal needle/hook

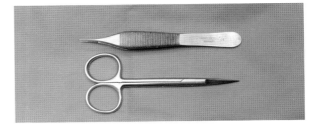

Figure 4-11. Forceps/scissors

stylet, the thread is inserted into the cannula; then, when the cannula is removed, the thread is left in place inside the skin. When using a thread that has been preloaded onto a needle, it is difficult to correct the position if the thread is placed incorrectly. However, when using a cannula, the position can be secured before inserting the thread, allowing more accurate thread placement while also reducing the risk of bruising.

5) Cannula/stylet/long needle (Figures 4–9, 4–10)

When using an anchoring thread, the thread needs to enter and then exit the skin. Here, a long needle can be used, passing the thread through the eye of the needle to allow it to be pulled back from the skin, or a cannula can be used as shown in the figure below.

6) Forceps/scissors (Figure 4–11)

These are used to hold or cut the thread.

SECTION 4

Design

Since the design depends heavily on the clinical appearance and individual circumstances of each patient, we will discuss the design later while looking at case studies.

SECTION 5

Anesthesia

The method of anesthesia can be determined according to the surgeon's convenience. Local anesthesia is most often used, as facial anesthesia is usually effective and does not cause any major problems during the procedure. However, procedural sedation is sometimes used due to the patient's psychological state or for other reasons. Local anesthesia can be broadly divided into mini tumescent anesthesia and nerve block.

1. Mini tumescent anesthesia

Mini tumescent anesthesia is a method adapted from the tumescent fluid technique used in liposuction, in which 2% lidocaine solution typically used for anesthesia is diluted to 1%

lidocaine solution (Tables 4-2, 4-3). The advantage of this solution is that pain is reduced when injected at the appropriate pH and bleeding tendency is minimized because epinephrine can help prevent bruising.

Nevertheless, the injection of a large volume of fluid can make swelling more severe, so patients should be thoroughly informed of this possibility. Moreover, solutions containing sodium bicarbonate can discolor when stored for a long time, so any remaining solution should be disposed after use. Typically, for facial anesthesia, 10 ㎖ of fluid is used per side, meaning that approximately 5 ㎖ of lidocaine is used in total.

Table 4-2. 1% lidocaine mini tumescent formula

Normal Saline : 60 ㎖
2% lidocaine : 60 ㎖
8.4% sodium bicarbonate : 12 ㎖
1:1000 Epinephrine : 1 ㎖

Table 4-3. 0.3% lidocaine mini tumescent formula

Normal Saline : 100 ㎖
2% lidocaine : 20 ㎖
8.4% sodium bicarbonate : 10 ㎖
1:1000 Epinephrine : 0.2 ㎖

2. Nerve block

Since nerve block is induced by generally well-known methods, we will omit a detailed explanation here (Figure 4-12).

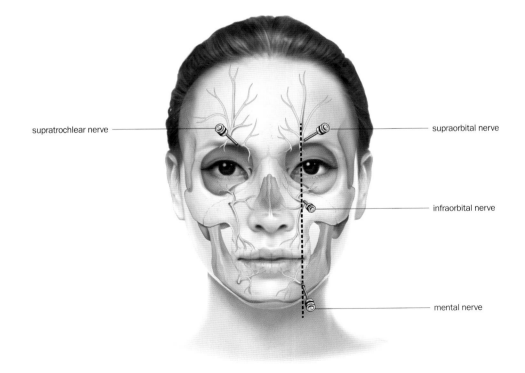

supratrochlear nerve

supraorbital nerve

infraorbital nerve

mental nerve

Figure 4-12. Typical nerve block locations

TEXTBOOK OF ABSORBABLE THREAD LIFTING

Chapter 05

Thread Lifting Techniques

SECTION 1

Thread Lifting Techniques: Non-barbed Thread Types and Techniques

The thread used in absorbable thread lifting can be broadly divided into non-barbed and barbed threads. Barbs can be made by physical manipulation of the thread or attachment of a specialized substance (e.g., barbs, mesh). Various types of non-barbed thread are used, and these are typically inserted into the subcutaneous soft tissue or muscle. For information about the characteristics of different thread materials, please refer to the sections above on types of thread.

1. Important factors when operating with monofilament thread

The most important factors when using a monofilament thread can be summarized with the acronym "DNDR" (Direction, Number, Depth, and Rotation).

1) Direction

Since collagen is produced in the direction orthogonal to the longitudinal axis of thread insertion, it is most effective to place the thread orthogonal to the intended lifting direction (Figure 5-1).

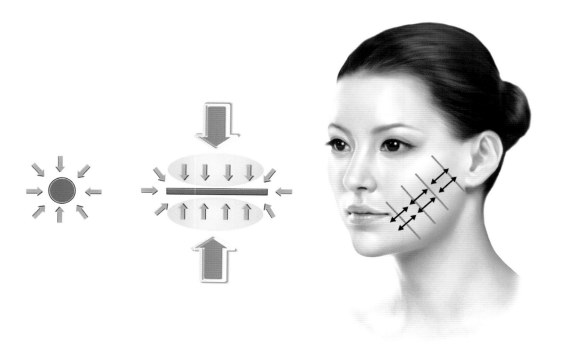

Figure 5-1. Blue, PDO thread; orange arrows, direction of tissue lifting; and red arrows, overall lifting direction

There is no objective or scientific basis for this direction, but our experience has shown far better results for this method compared to inserting the thread in the opposite direction (Figure 5-2).

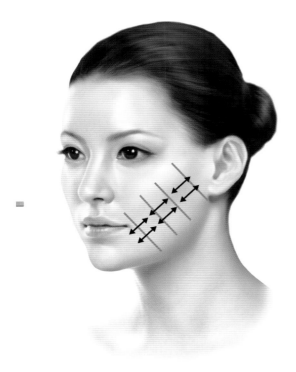

Figure 5-2. Direction of procedure for basic lifting

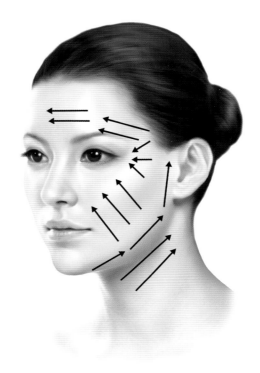

Figure 5-3. Overall direction and length of monofilament thread placement in the face

Ultimately, following this direction results in the thread being placed in the same orientation as that of face wrinkles, and this results in lifting orthogonal to the wrinkles, which produces a good outcome in most cases (Figure 5-3).

When using monofilament thread on the left cheek, the left hand is used to pull the cheek and jaw in the superolateral direction, and the thread is inserted from medial to lateral at intervals of approximately 1 cm (Figure 5-4). During thread insertion, it is important to use the left hand to ensure the depth of the needle is maintained directly below the dermis. Moreover, note that the first needle is not removed immediately after insertion, but all the needles are first inserted and then removed simultaneously. When operating on the right cheek, the same method is used, with the left hand gently pushing the right cheek in the superolateral direction (Figure 5-5).

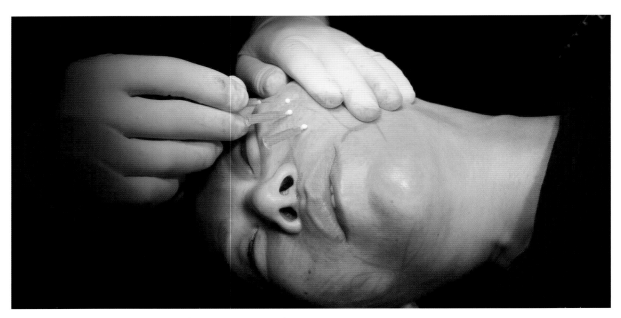

Figure 5-4. Technique for the left cheek (right-handed surgeon)

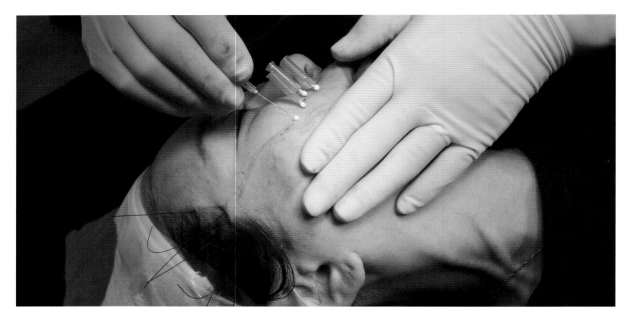

Figure 5-5. Technique for the left cheek (right-handed surgeon)

2) Number

Inserting a greater number of threads can provide greater skin regeneration effect via collagen stimulation, but inserting too many threads can lead to excessive bruising and edema. We recommend using approximately 50-100 threads throughout the entire mid- and lower face.

3) Depth

Although there may be a slight difference in depth depending on clinical indications, to induce collagen production, inserting the thread directly below the dermis is ideal.

If the aim of the procedure is fat loss, inserting the thread in the fat layer is better. When placing the monofilament thread, it is important to be careful not to place the thread too shallow. If the thread is placed superficial to the dermis layer, it can readily cause long-term problems such as a foreign body granuloma (Figure 5-6).

In this case, the best solution is to actively remove the thread. If that is not possible, in our experience, Hyalase (hyaluronidase) is more effective than triamcinolone injection. A more detailed discussion will be provided in the section on adverse effects.

4) Rotation

Typically, it is common to remove the needle directly after thread insertion, but we recommend rotating the needle at least 3-4 times immediately after insertion. This rotation can promote skin regeneration by aiding collagen production via mechanotransduction and also help the thread to grip the tissue internally.

When trying to remove the needle after insertion and rotation, the surgeon may feel the tissue holding onto the needle (needle grab phenomenon). The extent of this phenomenon varies according to the condition of the patient's tissue, and it is mostly experienced in younger patients with firmer skin. For this reason, it is acceptable to apply more rotation in older patients with slightly loose tissue (Figure 5-7).

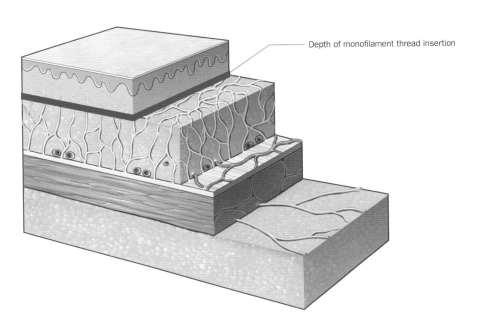

Depth of monofilament thread insertion

Figure 5-6. Cross-section of the skin

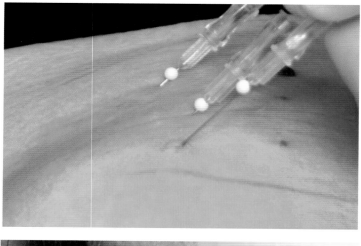

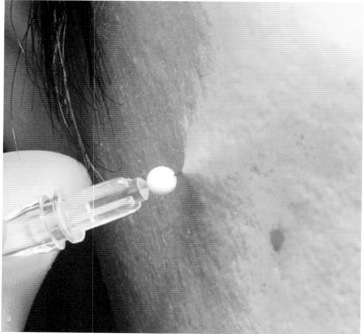

Figure 5-7. Changes in the skin immediately after rotating the monofilament thread (needle grab phenomenon)

2. Basic techniques using monofilament thread

For monofilament (plain/simple) thread, PDO is most often used. This thread has a smooth surface with no barbs. Although the thread is usually inserted in the hypodermis or subcutaneous fat layer, it can also be inserted in the muscle layer if necessary. After the procedure has been designed in the desired area, the thread is inserted using one of the several methods described below. The methods are categorized based on the passage of the needle through the soft tissue and muscle or by the layer in which the thread is placed.

1) Horizontal

In this method, the thread is inserted in a straight line, irrespective of whether the needle enters the skin orthogonally or at an angle. This is the most widely used method and usually involves the thread being inserted in parallel in the same subcutaneous layer (Figure 5-8).

2) Vertical

In this method, the thread is inserted orthogonally from the skin to the muscle. Usually, short monofilament threads of ≤2.5 cm are used. This method is generally used in reducing volume rather than lifting. Although the exact theory and background of this method are still unknown, we expect that volume reduction occurs because of muscle relaxation when the thread is placed in the muscle layer. This method is mostly used to reduce square jaws or large calves but can also be used in other areas, including the trapezius muscles (Figure 5-9).

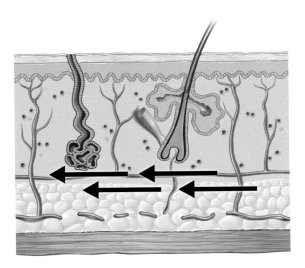

Figure 5-8. Horizontal technique

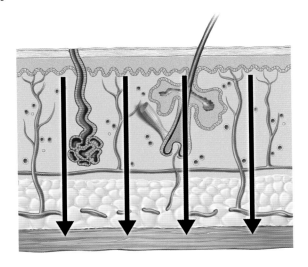

Figure 5-9. Vertical technique

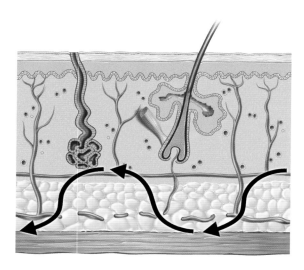

Figure 5-10. Sewing technique

3) Sewing

In this method, rather than inserting the thread at a constant subcutaneous depth, the thread is passed up and down, as if sewing, through multiple layers. This method has the effect of tightening several layers of loose tissue. It is mostly used to improve the jawline (Figure 5-10).

4) Zigzag

In this method, the thread is inserted in the same subcutaneous layer, moving side to side in a zigzag pattern. This is used to resolve deep wrinkles by bringing together the tissue on either side, such as in the correction of nasolabial folds or midcheek creases (Figure 5-11).

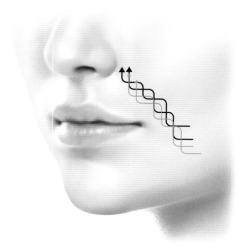

Figure 5-11. Zigzag technique

5) Circular

In this method, a circle is visualized around the area that needs correction, and multiple threads are inserted into the border of the circle, oriented toward the center (Figure 5-12).

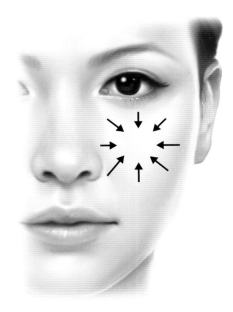

Figure 5-12. Circular technique

6) Framework (meshwork)

In this method, the thread is inserted in a grid pattern, in either the same subcutaneous layer or different layers. This is effective in compressing a thick tissue and reducing volume (Figure 5-13).

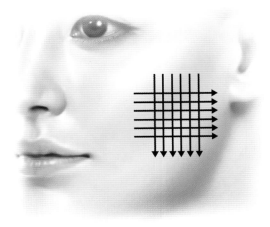

Figure 5-13. Framework technique

3. Clinical applications

Absorbable thread lifting has gained much popularity in only 3-4 years and is used in various fields of cosmetic surgery. However, there is still a lack of theoretical evidence, objective research, and precise treatment methods or their outcomes.

Even now, various animal experiments and clinical trials are being conducted for thread lifting, but unfortunately, objective proof has still not been demonstrated in academic publications. Since we feel that it is not appropriate to discuss theoretical evidence and experiments, we have instead chosen to focus more on practical and easy clinical applications.

In addition, there is still no consensus about standardized methods. We were unable to find any reference literature, and so we had to go through a long process of trial and error. For this reason, the methods presented in this book are based on shared opinions and techniques from our own experience and trial and error. It is possible that better methods exist, but we only present methods that are recognized to be safe, so we do not expect any of these methods to cause major problems.

Previously, in the field of dermatology, lifting was restricted to other methods, including the use of chemical substances for desquamation, which leads to increased elasticity during the regeneration process, and radiofrequency heat treatment or ultrasound to induce collagen synthesis. In the field of plastic surgery, facelift surgery is often performed, which simply removes the sagging skin.

We believe that absorbable thread lifting is an excellent new procedure to overcome the limitations of laser lifting in dermatology and facelift surgery in plastic surgery, while also maximizing the strengths of these procedures.

Thread lifting has been performed under various different names for approximately 10 years, including Aptos lift (Russia), contour thread (USA), and scaffold lifting. However, previous thread lifting methods typically used barbed thread, with the aim of physically pulling the sagging skin upward. In addition, because these procedures used non-absorbable thread, the thread remains permanently beneath the skin. This fundamental limitation makes any adverse events difficult to resolve and is a factor in the failure of such procedures to achieve widespread popularity.

Absorbable thread lifting, mostly using PDO thread, began to be performed in Korea from around 2010, overcoming some of the problems of previous thread lifting methods, and started to grow in popularity. Absorbable thread lifting can be considered to differ from previous non-absorbable thread lifting procedures in two aspects.

First, the biggest difference is that, rather than focusing simply on physical lifting of the skin, absorbable thread lifting simultaneously stimulates the tissue. This promotes regeneration of the dermis via collagen production and fibroblast proliferation, which results in increased skin elasticity.

Second, previous non-absorbable thread lifting techniques could cause nerve irritation or permanent asymmetry due to the remnant thread, and re-surgery was impossible. In contrast, for absorbable thread lifting, most adverse effects are temporary, and re-surgery is possible.

Here, we discuss various clinical applications using monofilament and cog threads.

1) Skin elasticity

Absorbable thread lifting is often used with the aim of improving skin elasticity, and in the early development of the procedure, this was the most common clinical indication. Usually, monofilament thread is used and placed at a depth directly below the dermis. A needle length of around 4 cm is suitable. The number of threads placed is equivalent to 50-100 threads for the whole midface and lower face area, which is the area typically targeted for lifting. We recommend inserting the thread orthogonal to the intended direction of lifting (Figure 5-14).

2) Jawline and double chin

The jawline, including a double chin, is one of the areas that patients most often want treated. The aims of treatment in this area are correction of so-called "marionette lines" (jowls) around the mouth, lifting of cheek tissue, increasing the elasticity of sagging skin around the jawline, and fat reduction below the jaw and around the mouth. The effect is usually increased by using monofilament and cog threads together (Figure 5-15).

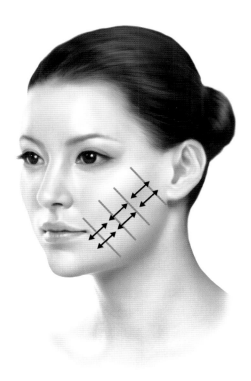

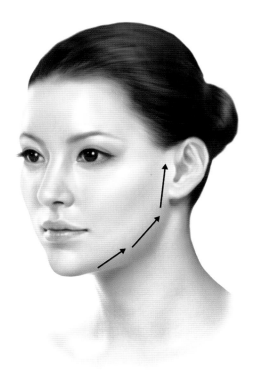

Figure 5-14. General direction of monofilament thread placement in procedures for skin elasticity

Figure 5-15. The placement of monofilament threads for jawline or double-chin correction

In operations on the jawline, it is common to use monofilament and cog threads in combination with two 17 (9)-cm floating bidirectional-type cog threads placed from the temple to the jowl and another two 17 (9)-cm floating bidirectional-type threads placed from the mastoid process behind the ear to the jowl. Here, it is important to be careful not to place the cog threads too deep because it can result in nerve injury. Next, the sewing technique is used to weave the monofilament thread through the fat layer, at a subdermal level, along the jawline. A thread length of 4-5 cm is appropriate, with about 20 threads being used per side (Figure 5-16).

In procedures to correct a double chin, the monofilament thread is placed at the subcutaneous level in order to remove the fat below the chin. Subject to the fat distribution under the chin, it is suitable to place 50-100 threads 3-4 cm in length. When cog thread is also used, two or three 17-cm floating bidirectional-type threads are placed from the mastoid process to midline beneath the chin. These threads are placed in the fat layer, slightly deeper than that in procedures to correct the jawline. The patient should be informed that the fat reduction effect is not immediate and usually becomes apparent after 1-2 months.

3) Nose

The first thread used for absorbable thread rhinoplasty in Korea was Misko. One of the authors (Chief Bong-Il Rho, Glovi Plastic Surgery Clinic) has been using Misko since participating as an early adopter; subsequently, various similar products have been developed and are being used. Fundamentally, only the cog thread is effective. Usually, this is used to lift

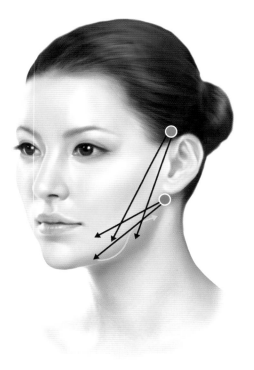

Figure 5-16. The technique combining monofilament thread and cog thread

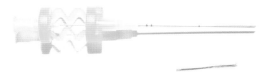

Figure 5-17. Misko thread

the nose tip but can also be used to raise the bridge and narrow the width and reduce the flare of the nasal area. The thread we use contains multidirectional cogs, and the end is frayed, which allows it to provide support without slipping on bone and also prevents the sharp thread end from penetrating the skin of the nose tip (Figure 5-17).

Before inserting the threads, an instrument such as that in the image below is used to pull the skin of the nose tip in the desired direction.

Cephalometric images can be used to compare the nose tip after lifting with cog thread to

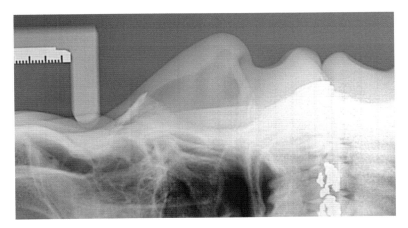

Figure 5-18. Preoperative cephalometry

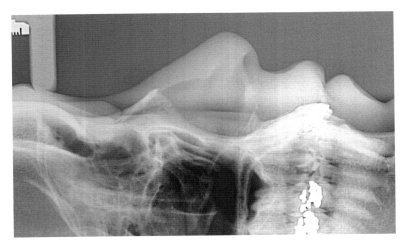

Figure 5-19. Postoperative cephalometry

confirm that it has been sufficiently lifted (Figures 5-18, 5-19). The procedure is simple and there is less swelling, making it suitable for patients with a high level of social activity. However, we do not believe that it can replace surgery.

Adverse effects include thread protrusion, scarring, and inflammation. Thread protrusion most commonly occurs at the site of insertion, and the major cause is that the thread was too long. In cases of intraoral thread protrusion, the thread needs to be removed. Rarely, scarring occurs at the site of thread insertion, and cases of inflammation are normally resolved by antibiotic medication.

4) Neck wrinkles

For neck wrinkle treatment, monofilament thread is better than cog thread. After marking the site of wrinkle formation preoperatively, 50-100 monofilament threads are inserted along the wrinkles at the subdermis level. We recommend placing 3-5 overlapping threads per wrinkle, using relatively short threads of 2.5-3 cm to account for the curve of the neck.

Unlike other areas, there is a high risk of bruising in the neck, and this should be made clear to the patient before the procedure. Better outcomes can be achieved by a combination with Botox or filler treatment (Figure 5-20).

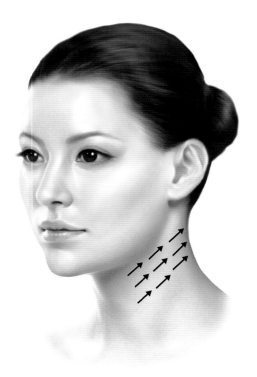

Figure 5-20. The technique for correcting neck wrinkles

5) Forehead wrinkles

In order to correct shallow forehead wrinkles, about 50 monofilament threads are placed along the direction of the wrinkles at the subdermis level. Like with neck wrinkles, 3-5 overlapping threads should be placed per wrinkle, using short threads 2.5-3 cm in length (Figure 5-21).

6) Eyebrow and forehead lifting

For forehead lifting, 6-7-cm-long thin 2-0 bidirectional cog threads are used and placed deep, directly above the periosteum, orthogonal to the forehead wrinkles, starting from 1-2 cm posterior to the hairline and extending toward the eyebrows. This ensures that the thread is not palpable or visible beneath the skin and also avoids irritation of the supraorbital and supratrochlear nerves. There are various techniques that can be used in this area, and with more experience, anchoring methods would also be worth trying (Figure 5-22).

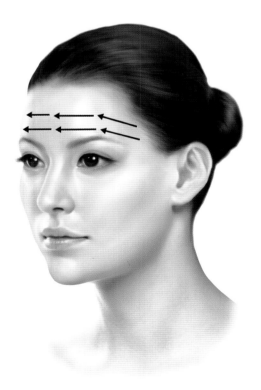

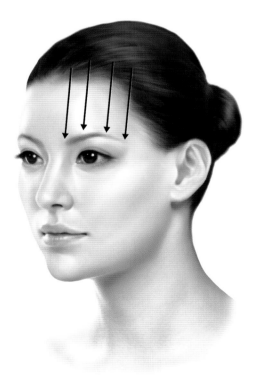

Figure 5-21. The technique for correcting forehead wrinkles

Figure 5-22. The technique for forehead lifting

7) Periocular region

① Crow feet

When operating to correct crow feet, the thread is placed along the wrinkles. In Botox therapy, the procedure is restricted to wrinkles at least 1 cm lateral to the lateral canthus, and smiling and other facial expressions may appear unnatural after treatment. By comparison, the advantages of thread lifting are that it is also able to improve wrinkles within 1 cm of the lateral canthus and does not lead to unnatural facial expressions. It is appropriate to use 10-20 short threads 2.5-3 cm in length per side, placing 2-3 overlapping threads per wrinkle. For crow feet, threads are sometimes placed in a meshwork pattern. Here, it is important not to insert the threads too superficially (Figures 5-23, 5-24).

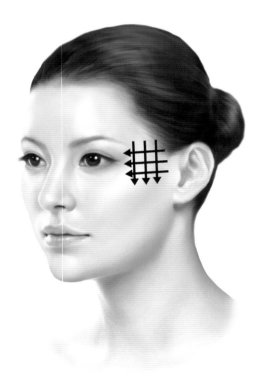

Figure 5-23. The periocular framework technique

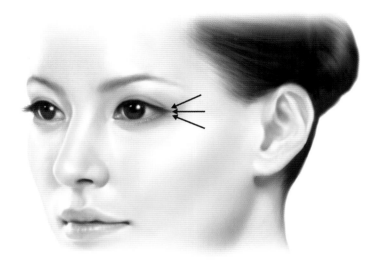

Figure 5-24. The technique for crow's feet correction

② Under-eye fine wrinkles

In treating fine wrinkles under the eye, approximately 10 short threads 2.5-3 cm in length are placed on each side. In our experience, we felt that the effect of thread lifting was slightly worse for under-eye fine wrinkles compared to other areas. We suspect that this is because the use of a needle causes relatively severe pain and bruising is readily induced even when using the smallest needle possible; these factors make it difficult to place a large number of threads below the eye. This leads to lower patient satisfaction, and ultimately, the discomfort may outweigh the effects (Figure 5-25).

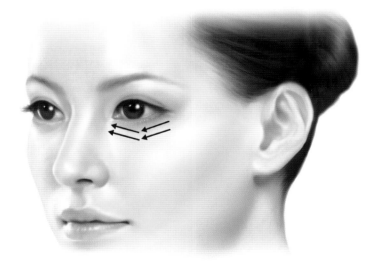

Figure 5-25. The technique for under-eye wrinkle correction

8) Nasolabial folds

For the nasolabial folds, 2-3 floating bidirectional cog threads 12-15 cm in length are placed at the depth of the SMAS along the trajectory of the zygomaticus minor muscle. In addition, 20 monofilament threads, per side, are placed in a zigzag pattern along the path of the nasolabial fold (Figure 5-26).

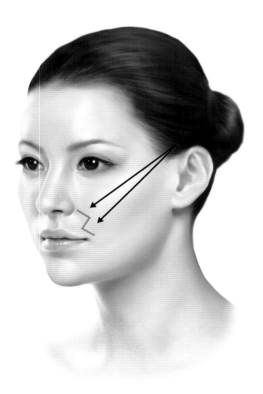

Figure 5-26. The technique for nasolabial fold correction

SECTION 2

Thread Lifting Techniques: Barbed Thread Types and Techniques

Now, we will discuss in detail the techniques using barbed thread.

Non-barbed thread lifting methods, in which threads are placed in various directions in different areas, are used frequently because the methods are simple and there is less swelling. However, these methods have small immediate lifting effect and poor effect persistence.

In order to maximize the lifting effect, it is necessary to use a thread that has been physically modified to contain barbs or cogs that can hook and raise the sagging tissue. There are several types of barbed thread that are categorized by the barb direction and use of anchoring. First, in terms of direction, they are classified as unidirectional thread, in which all the barbs face the same direction; bidirectional thread, with two sections of barbs facing opposite directions; and multidirectional thread, with multiple sections of barbs facing opposite directions. Barbed thread can then be further divided into anchoring-type or floating-type thread, depending on whether the thread is fixed after tissue lifting.

The most representative example of floating type thread is Aptos thread. These are bidirectional threads 7-10 cm in length, with barbs facing opposite directions in order to help the tissue gather at the center of the thread. This thread, developed by Russia's Dr. Sulamanidze, was made with non-absorbable polypropylene. However, recently, several products are being sold in Korea that use absorbable thread with a similar shape. These products also have bidirectional barbs that provide a lifting effect by causing the sagging tissue to gather at the center of the thread.

Although this is a familiar method that has been used for a long time, because the centers of the threads are located on the cheekbone, in Korean individuals, who often have well developed cheekbones, it can make the cheekbones more prominent.

Multidirectional cog threads were released to solve this problem; because the sagging tissue is not gathered at one specific location, the problem of making the cheekbones more prominent is reduced. However, the multidirectional thread is fundamentally different from the bidirectional thread; rather than generating a lifting effect by pulling tissues together, it acts as an anchor and is therefore better suited to be used in combination to boost the effects of the bidirectional thread, rather than as the only thread.

Typically, either the thread is inserted after placing an 18-G guide cannula, or like non-barbed thread, the thread that has been preloaded onto a needle can also be used.

1. Floating type

In this procedure, barbed thread is used to lift the sagging skin and tissue, but the thread is not tied or anchored anywhere. Typically, the bidirectional or multidirectional thread 7-15 cm in length is used.

Here, we discuss lifting procedures using floating-type thread, irrespective of the thread thickness or characteristics.

1) Thread characteristics

① Uni-directional thread

The unidirectional thread is available in various lengths. Because this thread cannot provide lifting simply by its presence, the ends of the threads need to be tied or looped together in order to produce a lifting effect (Figure 5-27).

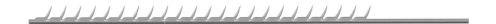

Figure 5-27. Unidirectional thread

② Bi-directional thread

This thread usually has a total length of 7-14 cm, and the barbed region has a length of 4-9 cm. Tissue is gathered toward the central area of the thread between the barbed regions. In individuals with prominent cheekbones, this thread has the disadvantage of making the cheekbones appear even larger.

The underlying principle of bidirectional thread lifting is that, when a force is applied, pulling loose and firm tissues together, the loose tissue moves toward the firm tissue. This is the reason why the skin on the lower face is pulled toward the temple when the bidirectional thread is inserted from the temple toward the lower face (Figure 5-20).

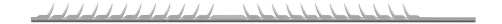

Figure 5-28. Bidirectional thread

③ Multi-directional thread

This thread usually has a total length of 7-14 cm, and the barbed region has a length of 4-9 cm. The thread contains bidirectional barbs in groups of 3-4, meaning that, unlike bidirectional thread, the thread secures the whole area, and the lifted tissue does not gather in a single location. Thus, this thread can be used in individuals with well-developed cheekbones.

However, since this thread provides fixation but does not lift up the tissue, it is used to strengthen anchoring after lifting the tissue with a unidirectional anchoring-type thread or bidirectional floating-type thread (Figure 5-29).

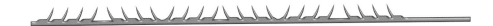

Figure 5-29. Multidirectional thread

Table 5-1. Types of cog thread by fixation type

Fixation type	Cog direction	Procedure characteristics	Strengths	Weaknesses	Diagram
Floating type	Uni-directional	Original procedure	Technical simplicity	No lifting effect	—
	Bi-directional	Most common	Lifting effect	Weaker than the anchoring type	Figure 5-32
	Multi-directional	Adjunctive	Strong anchoring	Difficult to use by itself	Figure 5-34
Anchoring type	Uni-directional	Classic method	Strongest lifting	Technical difficulty	Figure 5-31
	Bi-directional	Mixed procedure	Enables simultaneous lifting and fixation	Difficult to see the benefits of the anchoring point	Figure 5-33
Variant type	Uni-directional	Also referred to as soft anchoring	Effective lifting of small areas	Requires a process of knot tying and subcutaneous insertion	Figure 5-30

2) Instruments

Typically, a 17-19-G guide cannula is used to insert the thread. Since there is a high risk of bruising with even a slightly sharp tip, subject to the surgeon's preference, the procedure can be performed using a guide cannula with a blunt stylet. When selecting the guide cannula, the entire barbed region of the thread needs to be inserted under the skin, so the cannula should be at least 9 cm long.

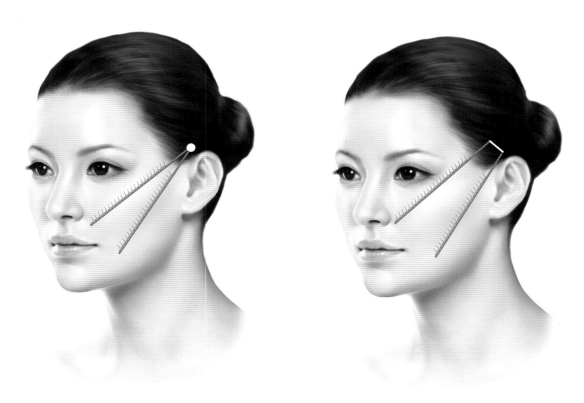

Figure 5-30. Variant (soft anchoring, tie) technique using unidirectional thread

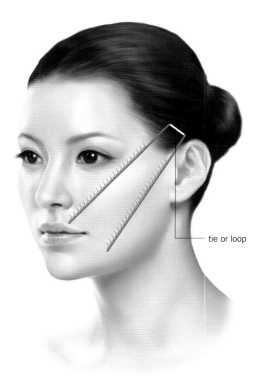

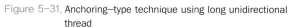

Figure 5-31. Anchoring–type technique using long unidirectional thread

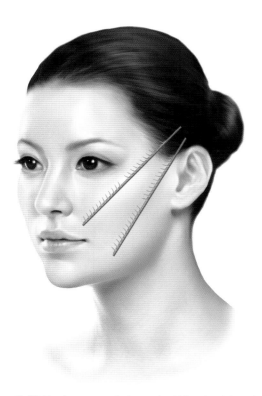

Figure 5-32. Floating–type technique using bidirectional thread

3) Design

The design will be discussed separately.

4) Anesthesia

Since a relatively large cannula is used, it is difficult to perform the procedure with topical anesthesia alone. Even if using procedural sedation, we also recommend using an injected anesthesia containing the vasoconstrictor epinephrine, in order to minimize the risk of bruising. Once familiar with the procedure, the pain under anesthesia is not too severe, so it is possible to perform the procedure with only local anesthesia.

The dilute tumescent fluid typically used in facelift surgery has a lidocaine concentration of 0.2-0.3% and epinephrine concentration of 1:250,000-500,000. With this in mind, a similar anesthesia solution can be injected in advance in the area where the cannula will be placed. Since there is a high likelihood of bleeding at the entry site, the epinephrine concentration is increased here.

We anesthetize the entry site with a solution that is commonly called dental lidocaine, containing 2% lidocaine and 1:100,000 epinephrine.

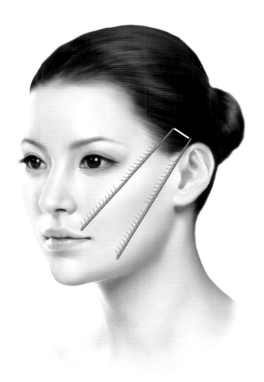

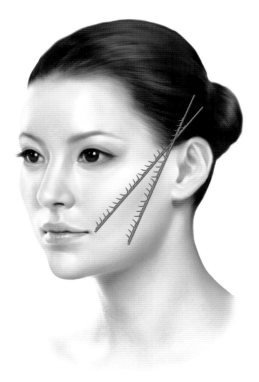

Figure 5-33. Anchoring-type technique using bidirectional thread

Figure 5-34. Floating-type technique using multi-directional thread

5) Surgical procedure

(1) An 18-G needle or awl is used to make an entry point in the designed location.

(2) The guide cannula is first inserted vertically and advanced to a depth depending on the subcutaneous fat layer. If the cannula is advanced too close to the surface, it can lead to postoperative skin crimping or dimples. Once the cannula has been inserted all the way, it is lifted gently toward the surface to determine the depth. If the cannula's shape is clearly visible or there is not a slight wobble, this means that the cannula has been placed too close to the surface. In this case, the guide cannula should be withdrawn slightly and reinserted.

(3) The stylet is removed, the thread is inserted via the cannula, and then the cannula is removed. Here, to avoid removing the thread, one hand is used to hold the thread in place, and the other hand is used to slowly remove the cannula. Once the cannula has been somewhat withdrawn, the end of the thread should be gripping the tissue, so the hand holding the thread can be removed and the cannula withdrawn fully.

(4) Once the thread is fixed, the thread protruding out of the skin is cut with scissors. If the thread is cut while gently pulling the thread and pushing on the skin on either side, the thread will naturally disappear beneath the skin after cutting.

(5) If a dimple is visible due to the dermis catching on the cut thread, this can be relieved by massaging.

SECTION 3

Thread Lifting Techniques: Anchoring Techniques

1. Background knowledge and basic principles

Anchoring techniques are effective thread lifting techniques for the significantly sagging skin or when a strong lifting effect is desired. Methods in which the thread is anchored superiorly can be categorized, according to the anchoring tissue, into classic-type (hard anchoring) methods, in which the thread is anchored to firm tissue such as the periosteum or deep fascia, and variant-type (soft anchoring) methods, in which the thread is anchored to a tissue with some mobility, such as subcutaneous fat, superficial fascia, or lower dermis.

Several anchoring techniques have been developed. In 2002, Dr. Gordon Sasaki published a paper on thread lifting method using Gore-Tex thread in Plastic and Reconstructive Surgery. This thread is commercially available in Korea, but the method is not used due to several associated issues. Thread lifting methods using a simple suture thread without any modifications have been used for a long time but never become popular.

Later, Russia's Dr. Sulamanidze developed a floating thread lifting method using barbed, non-absorbable thread. This was granted a global patent in 1999 and published in an academic paper in 2001, after which it became recognized and popular worldwide. This lifting method, using 10-cm-long bidirectional barbed thread is called the "Aptos (Anti-PTOSis) lift." However, surgeons became interested in anchoring techniques in order to further improve the lifting effect, and especially, methods using barbed, non-absorbable thread were developed and widely used.

The "classic-type" methods described here are techniques in which a thread is used to lift the sagging skin and anchored to firm tissue, such as the periosteum or deep fascia. These methods display the strongest lifting effects of all thread lifting techniques. However, due to the deep location of the anchoring tissue, a good knowledge of nearby anatomical structures is essential to minimize the adverse effects. Usually, these methods use long bidirectional thread of 40 cm or more in length, including a central region without bidirectional barbs.

However, recently, it has been possible to use a unidirectional thread with a looped end, by making a knot in the loop and anchoring the thread to the deep temporal fascia.

2. Main clinical indications

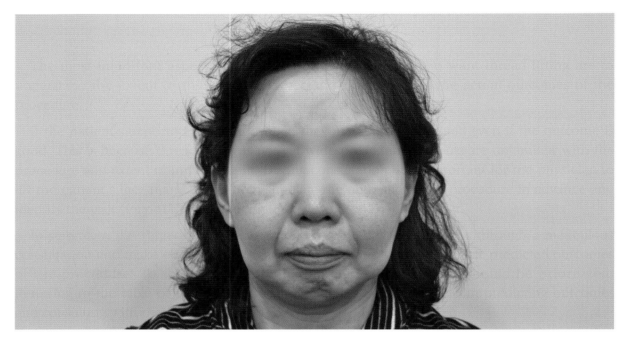

Figure 5-35. Preoperative photograph

1) Nasolabial folds

2) Sagging jowls

3) Sagging cheeks

4) Jawline improvement

5) Perioral wrinkle correction

3. Instruments

The instruments we generally use for thread lifting are anesthetic injections, an awl (to penetrate the skin), temporal needle, cannula, forceps, and scissors (refer to Chapter 4, p. 22). Depending on the type of thread, we use a 17-19-G guide cannula.

Figure 5-36. Image of unidirectional thread

4. Basic design

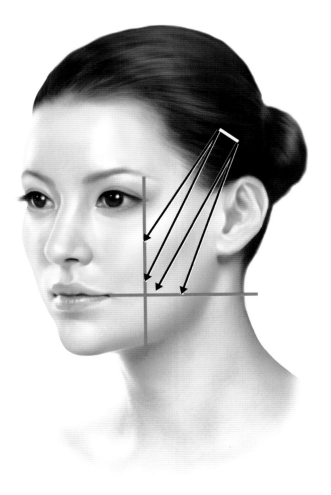

Figure 5-37. Basic design for the anchoring-type technique

1) In order to prevent visible protrusion of the thread during facial expressions or movement of the masseter muscle, a safe boundary is drawn (the red lines in the diagram). Inferiorly, the thread should not extend below the line connecting the oral commissure with the mandibular angle (horizontal red line). Medially, the thread should not extend beyond the line drawn directly downward from the lateral canthus (vertical red line).

2) The entry points for thread insertion are usually in the temporal region, 1-1.5 cm above the eyebrow, which is convenient for anchoring to the deep fascia and allows the cannula to be readily advanced to the desired area. The cannula exit point should be designed flexibly, within the safe boundary (red lines) as far as possible, according to the patient's

condition and location of the sagging skin.

3) For each side, at least 2 threads of 40 cm or longer are included in the design. The paths of the threads are marked according to the location of the sagging skin and the patient's desired lifting direction.

4) Specific designs

① Jawline (V-line)

Usually, this is a design to lift the sagging tissue in the cheek, making the face thinner and creating a so-called "V-line."

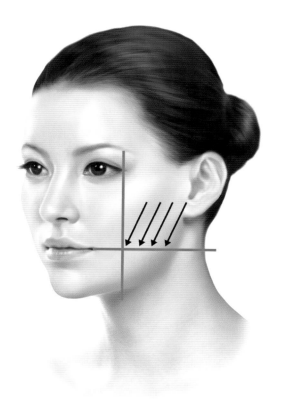

② Jowls

This is a design to lift the sagging skin next to the mouth.

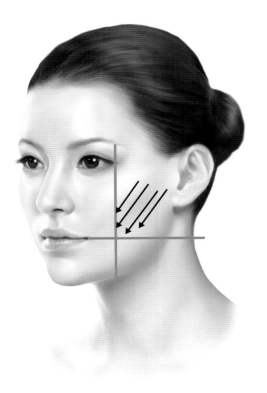

③ Nasolabial folds

This is a design to correct the nasolabial folds. Since this procedure can make the cheekbones appear wide, it should be designed with care for individuals who already have wide cheekbones.

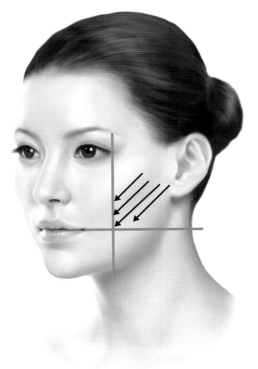

5. Surgical procedure

1) The surgical site is anesthetized. Usually, a 2% lidocaine solution containing 1:100,000 epinephrine is injected into the needle entry site, and mini tumescent solution is injected into the area of cannula passage, as described in the section on anesthesia. After the anesthesia injection, we recommend waiting for 5-10 min before beginning the operation, in order to prevent bleeding and bruising.

2) An 18-G needle or awl is used to pierce the skin at the site on the scalp. With experience, it is possible to use a temporal needle directly, without piercing the skin in advance. In order to prevent hair entering the hole, it is convenient to use an adhesive bandage to hold the hair out of the way or, as necessary, cut or shave the hair in this area prior to surgery.

3) The thread will be anchored in the deep temporal fascia. To ensure sufficiently deep anchorage in the deep temporal fascia, the needle is first inserted vertically until the surgeon encounters a bone-like structure. At this point, the round needle is rotated until it emerges through the scalp again. Care must be taken here since, if the thread is not

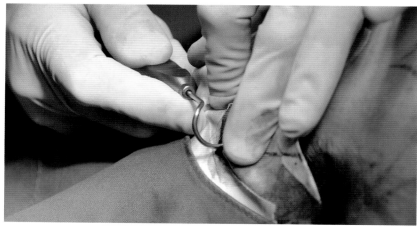

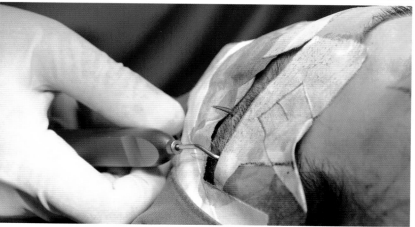

accurately anchored to the deep temporal fascia, the anchorage point can slip inferiorly, resulting in thread protrusion. In addition, if the loop moves inferiorly, it can damage the hair follicles, leading to hair loss.

4) After inserting one end of the thread into the hole in the temporal needle, the needle is rotated again to exit the scalp. Sometimes, two threads are inserted simultaneously, but depending on the direction of lifting, the anchor point may be changed, requiring the creation of more than two holes. The thread is adjusted so that it is of equal length on both sides, in order to position the center of the thread in the deep temporal fascia.

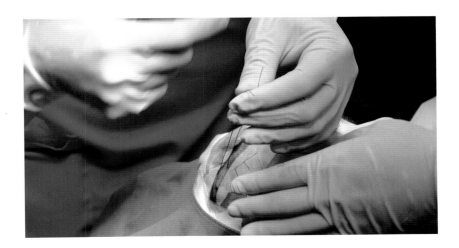

5) After inserting the cannula at the entry site, it is advanced toward the lower face at the depth of the deep subcutaneous fat layer, until it penetrates the skin again at the exit site. At this point, the cannula is not withdrawn but is positioned to span the entry and exit sites. When the cannula is inserted, it should be advanced with care while moving gently from side to side to avoid catching on the dermis; during this process, the cannula should be raised several times to check that it has not caught on the dermis.

6) Next, the thread is inserted into the cannula at the entry site and advanced to the end of the cannula at the exit site. Once the thread emerges at the exit site, the cannula is withdrawn via the exit site. When inserting the thread at the entry site, it is important to be careful not to let hairs enter the site. Any hairs that enter the site must be removed with forceps.

7) After inserting the thread on both sides, any thread protruding from the skin is cut and removed with scissors. It is necessary to pull the thread slightly during this process to prevent thread protrusion later during changes of facial expression.

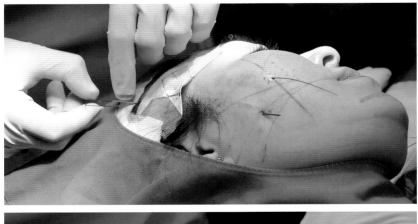

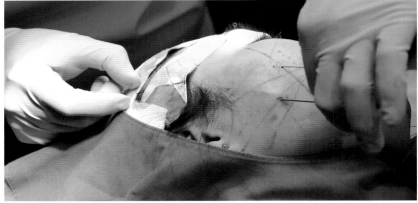

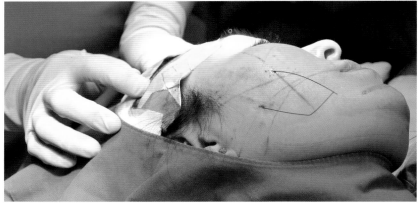

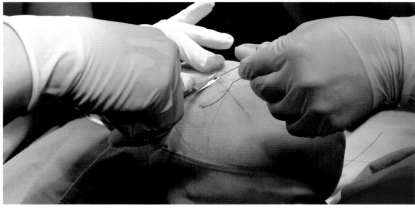

8) After removing the protruding thread, if there is any skin dimpling at the exit site, this can be alleviated by using one's hand to gently massage the affected area up and down. During massaging, it is common to hear popping sounds; this is not the thread snapping but a normal sound rising due to the release of tissue that had been caught on the barbs of the thread.

9) Before finishing the surgery, the patient's face is raised to the normal posture to check for symmetry and any adverse effects, such as dimpling.

6. Cautions

1) The patient may experience pain in the area of surgery for 1-2 postoperative weeks. During this time, it is important to prescribe the necessary medication and warn patients to avoid excessive use of the facial muscles or opening their mouth too wide.

2) Although the skin around the cheekbones may appear swollen postoperatively, this resolves naturally within 2-3 weeks on average.

3) Due to the effects of partial anesthesia during surgery, the patient may complain of discomfort opening or closing their eyes immediately after surgery or show unnatural movements of the perioral muscles as if the mouth has receded. These effects will disappear within approximately one day, so patients should be given a thorough explanation in advance to prevent undue concern.

4) The most important thing to pay attention to during the course of postoperative monitoring is skin dimpling at the exit site. If there is any skin dimpling, this needs to be actively resolved. If this goes unresolved for more than 4 weeks, it can result in a permanent dimple. Since there are cases of skin dimpling that go unnoticed by the patient, if possible, it is important to ensure that the patient returns for monitoring after 3-4 weeks and to observe the patient carefully.

7. Pre- and postoperative clinical photographs

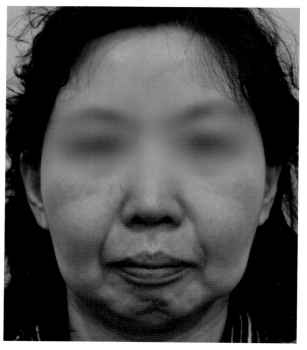 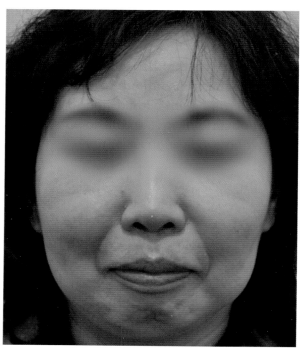

Figure 5–38. Pre– and postoperative photographs (front)

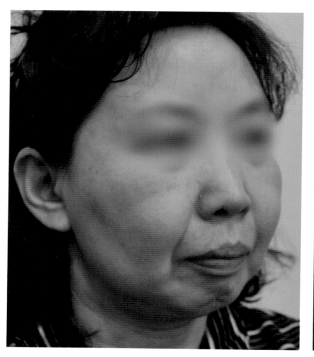 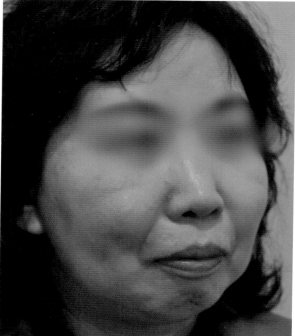

Figure 5–39. Pre– and postoperative photographs (right side)

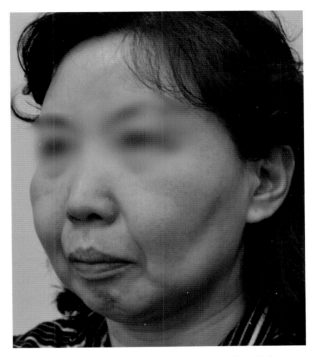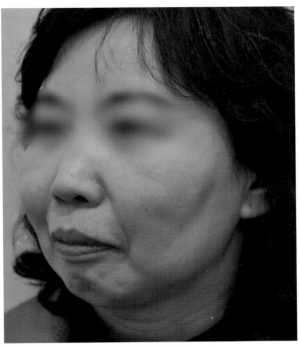

Figure 5-40. Pre- and postoperative photographs (left side)

[References]

1. (Meloplication of the Malar Fat Pads by Percutaneous Cable-Suture Technique for Midface Rejuvenation: Outcome Study(392 Cases, 6 Years' Experience). Plastic & Reconstructive Surgery. 09/2002: 110(2):635-54)

2. (Facial lifting with APTOS threads. Int J Cosmetic Surg Aethetic Dermatolo 2001;4:275-281)

SECTION 4

Thread Lifting Techniques: Variant Techniques

1. Background knowledge and basic principles

We use the term "variant type" (or "soft anchoring") to refer to methods of anchoring absorbable thread to somewhat mobile tissue, such as subcutaneous fat, superficial fascia, and lower dermis. Usually, a unidirectional thread is used and anchored to the tissue with a knot, so this technique is also called the "tie technique."

Compared to anchoring techniques, the base of support is relatively weak, but the procedure can be used in smaller areas; it is technically simpler; there is no need to remove hairs from the area; and common side effects of anchoring techniques, such as headache, can be avoided. Moreover, anchoring techniques often cause the cheekbones to appear larger; this is not a problem in variant techniques, and the considerable reduction in swelling and bleeding immediately after surgery allows patients to see the outcomes instantly.

2. Main clinical indications

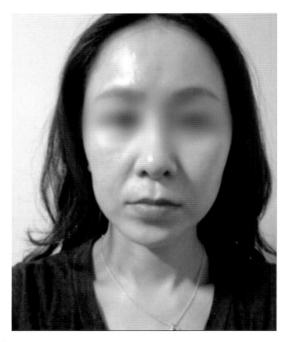

Figure 5–41. Preoperative photograph

1) Large cheekbones

2) Dimples beneath the cheekbones

3) Thin face (hollow cheeks)

4) Sagging jowls

5) Sagging cheeks

6) Jawline correction

7) Desiring surgery for only part of the face

8) Desiring a rapid recovery

3. Instruments

1) Absorbable unidirectional thread

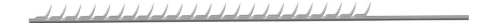

Figure 5-42. Image of unidirectional thread

2) Blunt cannula and anesthetic cannula (liposuction cannula or microcannula used in filler procedures)

3) Anesthesia solution 10-20 ccmL

⟨50 years old: bupivacaine 20 mL + epinephrine 0.3 ccmL

≥50 years old: Naropinropivacaine 20 mL + epinephrine 0.3 ccmL

4) Dental lidocaine - perioral anesthesia

5) 18-G needle (for entry site puncture)

4. Basic design

The entry sites are located superiorly, where a line drawn horizontally from the eyebrow meets the hairline, and inferiorly, on the hairline at a point 1 cm above the superior margin of the tragus. The trajectories of the threads can be designed based on the intended lifting direction (Figures 5-43, 5-44).

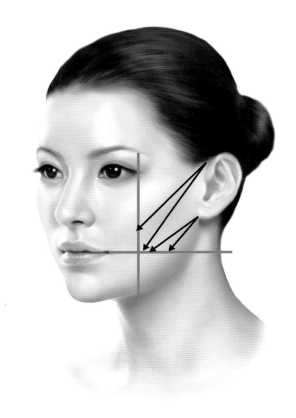

Figure 5-43. Basic design for the variant technique

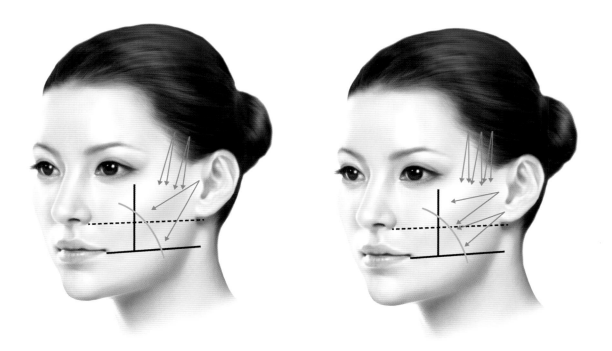

Figure 5-44. Sample clinical design for the variant technique

After tying a knot between the two threads, if the angle between the threads is too small, the tension can cause the knot to cut into the tissue and descend. For this reason, the angle between the two threads should be maintained at approximately 45°.

5. Surgical procedure

1) Dental lidocaine is used as entry site anesthesia.

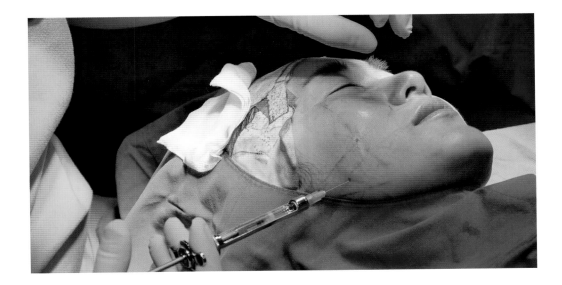

2) In order to secure a hole for the knot to enter, a small incision is made with a No. 11 scalpel or the skin is punctured with an 18-G needle.

3) Anesthesia is applied on the path of the thread using a guide cannula or a 23-G needle.

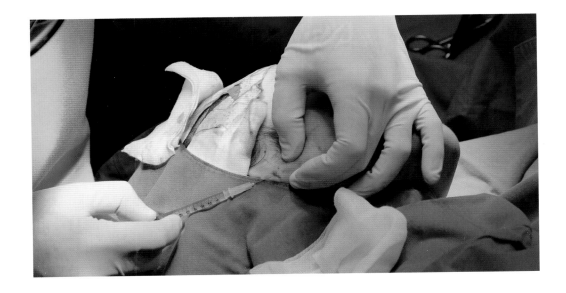

4) Generally, at least 4 unidirectional threads 10 cm or longer are prepared.

5) While pinching the skin so that it rises slightly with one hand, the other hand is used to insert a blunt cannula and advance it to the depth of thread placement in the subcutaneous fat layer. The cannula does not penetrate the skin.

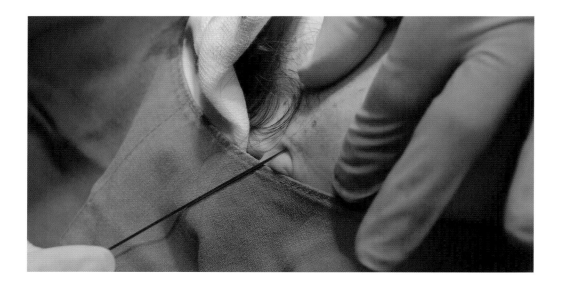

6) After stroking the thread to check that the cog direction is from the cannula entry site to the tip, the thread is inserted to the end of the cannula. While holding the thread with one hand, the other hand is used to gradually withdraw the cannula, leaving only the thread anchored beneath the skin.

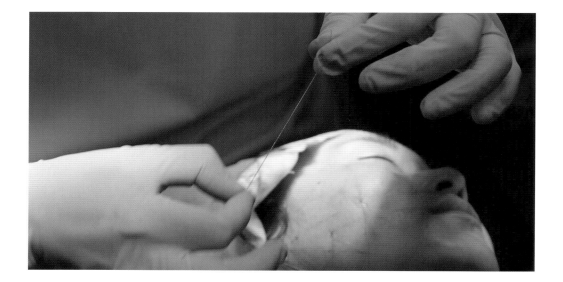

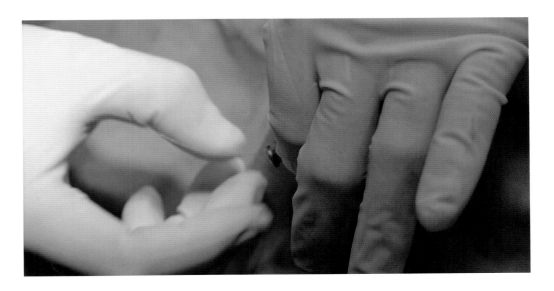

7) The cannula is inserted along the designed path for the thread in the same entry site.

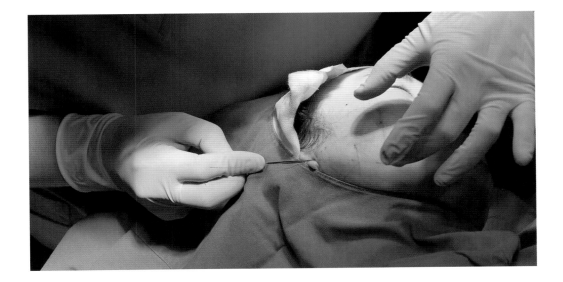

8) The guide stylet is removed.

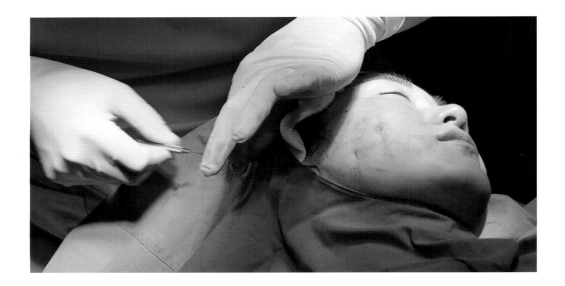

9) As in step 6), the thread is inserted, and the cannula is withdrawn.

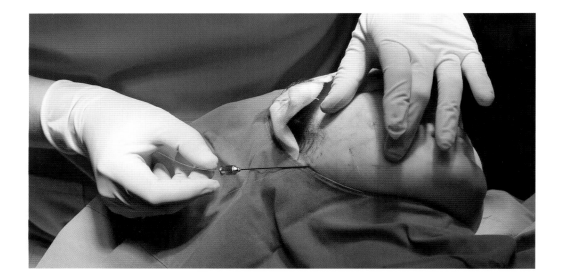

10) The two threads emerging from the same hole are tied at least 3 times (tie method).

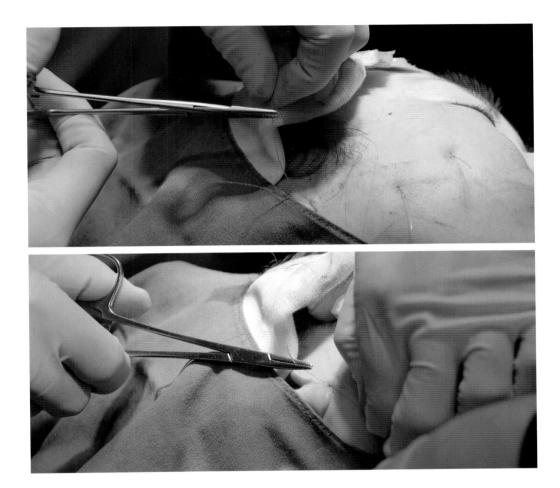

11) The thread is cut as close to the knot as possible.

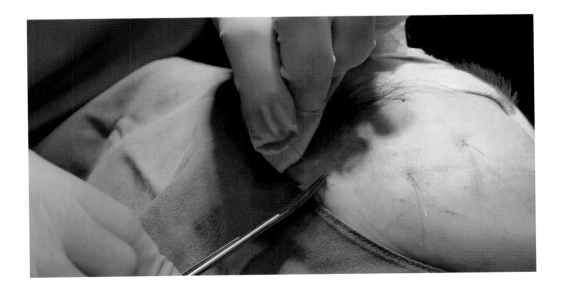

12) After the knot has been positioned beneath the skin, the surgery is completed (the knot can be pushed under the skin with forceps or scissors).

13) No special dressing is required postoperatively.

6. Cautions

1) The patient may experience pain in the area of surgery for 1-2 postoperative weeks. During this time, it is important to prescribe the necessary medication and warn patients to avoid excessive use of the facial muscles or opening their mouth widely.

2) The skin near the site where the thread was tied may appear swollen, but this usually resolves naturally after 2-3 weeks.

3) Due to the effects of partial anesthesia during surgery, the patient may complain of discomfort opening or closing their eyes immediately after surgery or show unnatural movements of the perioral muscles as if the mouth has receded. These effects will disappear within approximately one day, so patients should be given a thorough explanation in advance to prevent undue concern.

4) The most important aspects to pay attention to during the course of postoperative monitoring are pain and skin dimpling on the site where the threads were tied. If there is any skin dimpling, this needs to be actively resolved. If this goes unresolved for more than 4 weeks, it can result in a permanent dimple. Since there are cases of skin dimpling that go unnoticed by the patient, if possible, it is important to ensure that the patient returns for monitoring after 3-4 weeks and to observe the patient carefully.

7. Pre- and postoperative clinical photographs

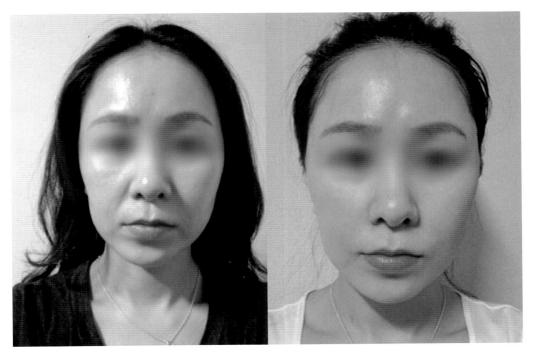

Figure 5-45. Frontal photograph after 1 postoperative week

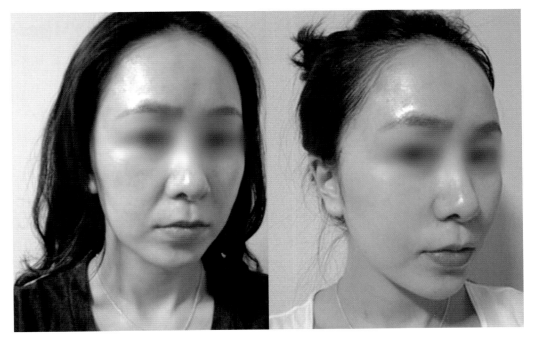

Figure 5-46. After 1 postoperative week

SECTION 5

Thread Lifting Techniques: Floating Techniques

1. Background knowledge and basic principles

In non-barbed thread lifting techniques, threads are positioned in various directions and locations in order to improve skin elasticity and provide a lifting effect. These methods are commonly used because they are technically easy and cause less swelling. However, these techniques have from limited immediate lifting effect on sagging tissue and poor effect persistence.

In order to achieve a better lifting effect, it is necessary to use a thread that has been physically modified to contain barbs or cogs.

In barbed thread lifting, a barbed thread is inserted in the sagging skin or subcutaneous tissue, and after pulling this tissue in the desired direction, the thread is anchored. In this section, we discuss floating-type techniques, in which thread fixation is achieved by the forces from the actual barbs, rather than making a physical anchor point in the skin or subcutaneous tissue.

The most well-known thread in floating-type techniques is the Aptos thread. This thread, developed by Russia's Dr. Sulamanidze, is a barbed thread made from non-absorbable polypropylene, with a length of 7-10 cm. The barbs face from the ends of the thread toward the center, so when the thread is placed within the skin or subcutaneous tissue, the tissue gathers at the center of the thread.

Recently, with an increase in the use of PDO, a number of PDO threads with various lengths and barb shapes have become commercially available. Currently, the most commonly used type is the bidirectional cog thread, in which the barbs are facing each other.

This thread also causes the tissues to gather at the center of the thread, like the Aptos thread mentioned above; the procedure is relatively simple, but the anchor point can be made in various locations, enabling lifting in the desired direction, and the lifting effect is relatively strong, making this one of the most widely used basic thread lifting methods.

The principle of bidirectional thread lifting is that when a force is applied between the firm and flexible tissues, the flexible tissue is pulled toward the firm tissue. Thus, when the firm temporal region is connected by a thread to the flexible skin of the lower face, the tissue of the lower face is pulled toward the temporal region.

The advantages of this method, compared to anchoring-type techniques, are as follows: there is less restriction on the number of threads, the procedure is simpler, there is less postoperative pain in the temporal region, and recovery is faster.

The threads used in this procedure include the bidirectional barbed thread; multidirectional cog/zigzag cog thread, which contains several repeating sections of bidirectional barbs; and spike cog thread, which contains barbs on the upper and lower parts of the thread facing opposite directions (Figure 5-47).

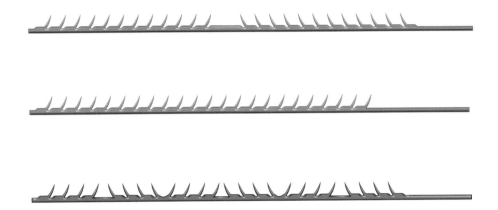

Figure 5-47. Various threads

2. Main clinical indications

The main clinical indications for which this procedure is performed are listed below:

1) Jowls

2) Nasolabial folds

3) Jawline correction (V-line)

4) Double chin

5) Overall lifting/elasticity enhancement

6) Eyebrows/forehead

3. Instruments

1) Design: Surgical marker pen, board marker pen, and pencil

The design is drawn using commonly used surgical marker pens, other marker pens, or pencils used for filler procedures. Surgical marker pens are difficult to erase, which makes them convenient during surgery, but can remain postoperatively. For this reason, board marker pens are commonly used.

2) Hair tidying: Hairband, elastic band, and tape

With floating-type thread lifting techniques, it is rarely necessary to cut the hair. However, if hair enters the skin, it can cause inflammation and a foreign body reaction subsequently, so it is important to be careful to keep hair out of the surgical site. To minimize the risk, it is helpful to use a hairband or elastic band to secure any hair near the surgical site and attach a tape along the hairline to reduce contact with hair.

3) Sterilization: Povidone iodine, chlorhexidine, sterilization drapes, and surgical drapes

The surgical site should be thoroughly sterilized to prevent infection. Generally, povidone iodine or chlorhexidine, which are used for injections, can be used to sterilize the surgical site. In particular, due to the possibility of contact with hair during the procedure, we recommend sterilizing the scalp as far as possible, including any taped areas, beyond the immediate surgical site. Subsequently, sterilized drapes should be used to ensure that only the surgical site is exposed.

4) Anesthesia: 2% lidocaine, normal saline, epinephrine, and sodium bicarbonate

Since a relatively wide cannula or long needle is used during the procedure, in most cases, topical anesthesia alone is insufficient. In addition, bruising often occurs when the procedure is performed using a needle, so to minimize this risk, an anesthetic injection containing the vasoconstrictor epinephrine can be administered preoperatively.

At the entry site, a needle or awl is used to penetrate the skin and insert the thread, so we recommend first administering an anesthetic injection in this area; typically 1-2% lidocaine solution containing 1:100,000 epinephrine is used. Because lidocaine is acidic, including 8.4% sodium bicarbonate in the anesthetic solution can help to reduce the pain associated with anesthesia.

Next, an anesthetic injection is applied on the area where the thread will be placed finally. Generally, the tumescent solution used in facelift surgery is prepared with 0.2-0.3% lidocaine and 1:250,000-500,000 epinephrine. However, the anesthetic solution that we use is shown below. The solution is applied using a 26-30-G long needle or cannula. For the bidirectional thread, the length of the barbed section is usually around 9 cm, so we use an anesthetic cannula with an internal diameter of 0.7-0.8 mm and a length of approximately 10 cm. To reduce the risk of bruising, it is helpful to wait for 5 min after anesthesia administration before beginning the surgery.

Anesthetic solution

N/S 100 mL   2% lidocaine 20 mL

8.4% sodium bicarbonate 10 mL   1:1,000 epinephrine 0.2 mL

5) Thread

Currently, the barbed thread is sold either in a package containing only the barbed thread or preloaded into a needle or cannula. When using a cannula in the procedure, the needle attached to the thread is not necessary, so if a preloaded thread is used, this will require an additional process of removing the thread from the needle. If there is a segment at the ends of the thread without barbs, scissors are used to cut off the part without barbs, making sure that the ends of the thread are barbed.

6) Cannula

In order to reduce bruising and tissue damage during the procedure, we recommend using a blunt cannula over a sharp needle. Recently, products are available with the thread and cannula as one; these products can be used, or the cannula can be prepared separately.

If the cannula is to be prepared, the internal diameter and length need to be decided. For standard barbed thread with a thickness of 1-0 or 2-0, an 18-G or 19-G cannula, respectively, can be prepared. However, when using the molding-type barbed threads or the threads with deeper barbs that are being made recently, the internal diameter of the cannula needs to be one grade wider (1-0, 17G; 2-0, 18G).

Since the length needs to include the entire barbed section, we suggest checking the length of this section on the thread that will be used and using a cannula that is 0.5-1 cm longer (for 9 cm cog thread, use a cannula with a length of 9.5-10 cm).

4. Basic design

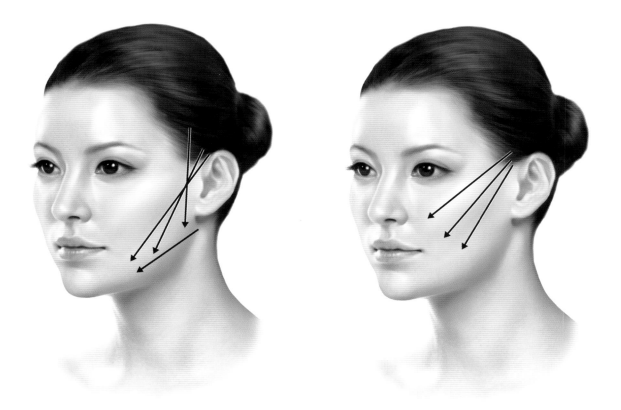

Figure 5–48. Basic design for the floating technique (left) for large and (right) small cheekbones

5. Surgical procedure and minimizing adverse effects

1) Using a cannula

(1) An 18-G needle or awl is used to penetrate the skin at the designed entry site. We recommend using an awl over a needle, since the risk of vascular injury is lower.

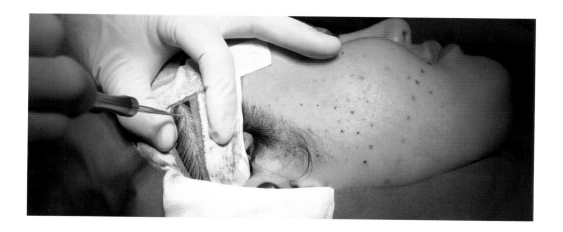

(2) First, the cannula is inserted vertically. Once the cannula has been inserted at the depth of the subcutaneous fat layer or just before the fascia, the cannula is rotated 90° and moved in the subcutaneous tissue until it is parallel to the skin. For right-handed surgeons, the cannula usually will be controlled by the right hand; in this case, the left hand can be used to raise the skin in the projected path of the cannula, which helps to ensure that the cannula is located in the subcutaneous fat layer and follows the appropriate trajectory.

If the cannula is inserted too deep, it can cause damage to other tissues, such as the salivary glands; if it is too shallow, there is a risk of skin crimping or dimpling. The intended depth is the subcutaneous fat layer. Once the cannula has been inserted fully, it can be raised toward the surface to estimate the depth. If the shape of the cannula is clearly visible or a slight wobble cannot be observed, the cannula has been inserted too close to the surface; in this case, the cannula should be removed and re-inserted in the subcutaneous layer.

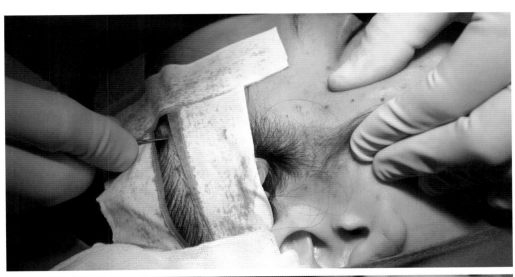

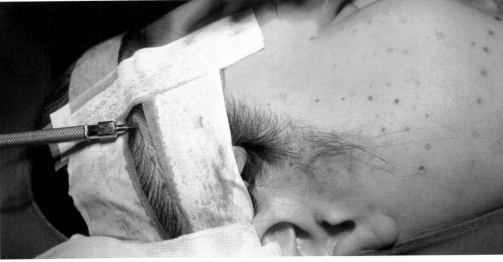

(3) After removing the stylet from the cannula, the thread is placed inside the cannula. The thread is introduced until the barbed section has been fully inserted and the thread cannot be advanced any further. For right-handed surgeons, the cannula can be withdrawn slowly using the left hand while the right hand continues to push the thread; this allows the barbs at the end of the thread to anchor to the skin. Once the cannula has been withdrawn 1-2 cm, the thread is pulled with the right hand to check for anchorage before removing the rest of the cannula.

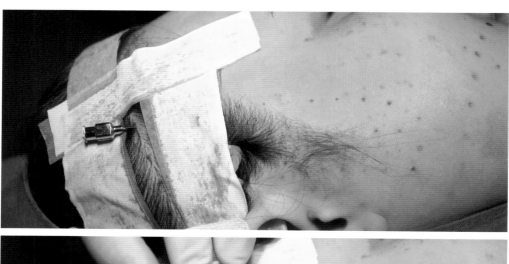

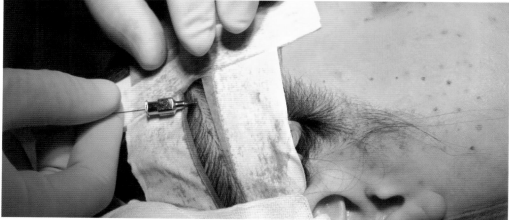

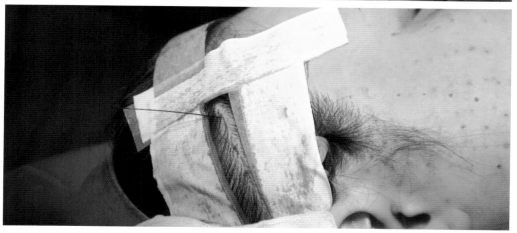

If the thread is not anchored and is pulled out, because the barbs at the end of the thread did not come in contact with the subcutaneous tissue, the procedure can be repeated using the same method. If thread anchoring fails continually, first check that there are barbs at the end of the thread, inspect the inside of the cannula for any obstructions, and check that the thread is not bending during insertion. If anchoring still fails, the procedure should be repeated using a new thread.

(4) After performing the thread lifting procedure as described above, the patient is lifted into a sitting position to adjust left-right symmetry. If one side is lifted more compared to the other, adjustments can be made by further inserting or pulling the thread on that side.

(5) Once symmetry has been confirmed, the thread protruding from the skin is cut using scissors. While cutting, the thread should be pulled slightly with one hand, and the scissors should be pushed gently toward the skin. This causes slight skin dimpling at the entry site, but if the thumb is placed slightly distal to the dimpling and a force is applied in the proximal direction, the skin dimpling disappears, and the thread is positioned beneath the skin.

If the thread is strongly pulled, the barbs that need to support the tissue can be lost, resulting in movement of the thread. Therefore, the surgeon should be careful not to strongly pull the thread during cutting.

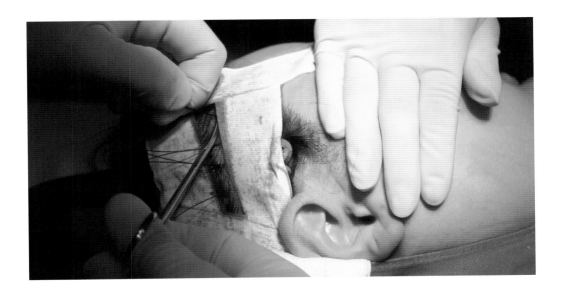

2) Using an all-in-one needle/cannula + barbed thread

The basic technique is the same as that using a cannula, but in using an all-in-one product, once the needle or cannula has been inserted into the subcutaneous tissue, it cannot be corrected, so it needs to be inserted at the correct depth. For this reason, we only recommend using this method after familiarizing the method using a cannula.

3) Advanced tips to reduce adverse effects

(1) Tips to avoid skin dimpling and thread migration

Skin dimpling refers to the condition where the skin being pulled by the thread collapses, like a dimple. Skin dimpling can sometimes be left deliberately in order to enhance the immediate postoperative lifting effect and occur belatedly after 1-2 postoperative weeks. If skin dimpling occurs, it should be actively resolved as soon as possible. Since it can be difficult to resolve after 1 month, due to adhesion, dimpling should ideally be resolved within 1 postoperative month. Skin dimpling usually disappears with firm massaging in the opposite direction to the barbs within 3-4 postoperative weeks. Since there may be pain during this procedure, local anesthetic injections can be administered. If massaging does not eliminate any skin dimpling, the thread should be removed.

When using a barbed thread, the thread can migrate superiorly or inferiorly, causing it to bulge like a pimple. This occurs when the thread anchorage is too weak to counter the forces tending toward migration in the opposite direction. If bidirectional barbed thread is being used, it is important not to damage the barbs, and the thread should be inserted such that the length of thread with barbs in each direction is similar. If the end of the thread is protruding like a pimple, an 18-G wide needle can be used to penetrate the skin, and microforceps or a similar instrument can be used to pull out the thread. If the thread needs to be removed, do not cut and partially remove it – it must be removed completely. During changes in facial expression, such as smiling, mastication, or speaking, the zygomaticus major muscle contracts, and if the

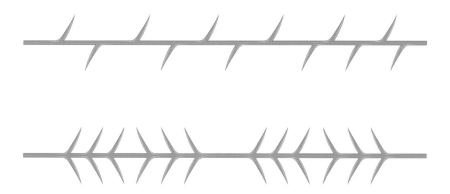

Figure 5-49. Threads that perform an anchoring role

end of the thread catches near the surface of the skin, it can cause dimpling. If barbs in the anchored part of the thread are weak or come undone, the thread can migrate inferiorly within the face or protrude. As mentioned above, compared to bidirectional barbed thread, zigzag or spike cog thread, due to its structure, is weaker at gathering tissue in one place, which leads to a reduced lifting effect. However, the advantage of this thread is that it results in less migration. Therefore, when performing floating-type thread lifting, using a combination of this thread with bidirectional barbed thread can help prevent adverse effects such as skin dimpling. Based on our experience, we use a 1:1 combination of bidirectional barbed thread and a thread that can fulfill an anchoring/support role (Figure 5-49).

(2) Tips to prevent cheekbones to appear larger – using short bidirectional barbed threads

The most commonly used bidirectional threads at present usually have a barbed length of about 9 cm. Bidirectional thread gathers tissue toward the central section between the sets of opposing barbs, but when the barbed section is 9 cm long as with the most commonly used bidirectional barbed threads, since the thread is placed 1-2 cm above the eyebrows down to the jawline, the central region between the barbs, unfortunately, ends up near the cheekbone, which makes it difficult to avoid the cheekbones appearing larger after the procedure. This phenomenon can be reduced using short bidirectional barbed threads, in which the barbed section is around 6 cm long, positioned from the hairline at the height of the lateral canthus in a vertical direction toward the jawline. Since the shorter barbed length results in a weaker grip on the skin tissue, it is important to use a thread that can hold the skin firmly. Generally, molding-type thread over cutting-type thread, a greater number of barbs per unit area, and bidirectional thread over unidirectional thread attach more strongly to the skin; this should be taken into account when selecting the thread to be used (Figures 5-50, 5-51).

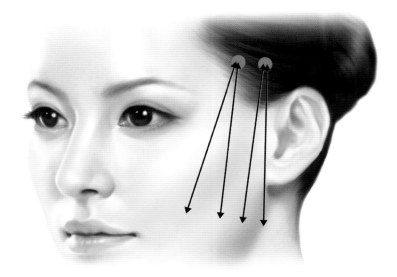

Figure 5-50. Design using standard bidirectional barbed thread

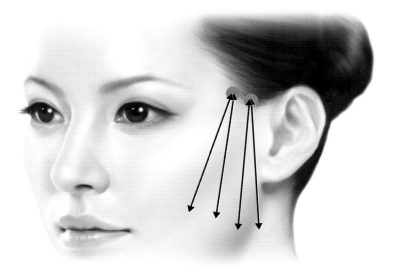

Figure 5-51. Design using short barbed thread

6. Cautions

1) The patient may experience pain after floating-type thread lifting surgery for 1-2 postoperative weeks, especially near the entry site or where the barbs of the thread touch the skin. Since irritation, such as pressing the surgical site or opening the mouth widely, can make the pain more severe, patients should be instructed to avoid excessive use of their facial muscles and not to open their mouth too wide.

2) The skin near the cheekbones may appear swollen after surgery, but this usually resolves naturally after 2-3 weeks.

3) Due to the effects of partial anesthesia during surgery, the patient may complain of discomfort opening or closing their eyes immediately after surgery or show unnatural movements of the perioral muscles as if the mouth has receded. This should be explained to the patient in advance.

4) During the first postoperative month, skin dimpling can occur. If this persists beyond the first postoperative month, it can result in a permanent dimple. Therefore, if skin dimpling is observed, it should be actively resolved as soon as possible.

7. Pre- and postoperative clinical photographs

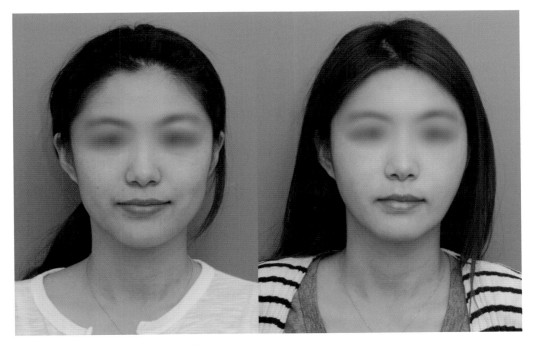

Figure 5-52. Frontal view after 3 postoperative months

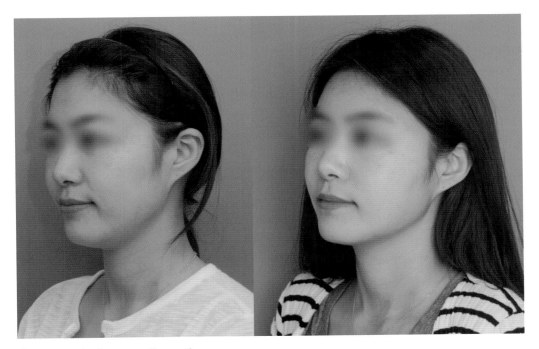

Figure 5-53. Side view after 3 postoperative months

SECTION 6

Thread Lifting Techniques: Vertical Lifting Techniques

1. Background knowledge and basic principles

In facial aging, the effects of gravity and loss of collagen from the skin cause the skin to descend vertically. During this process, various retaining ligaments form the structures supporting the tissue. As a result, the sagging skin shows an inferomedial pattern, gathering around the jowls (marionette lines). For this reason, lifting therapy has focused strictly on lifting in the opposite, superolateral direction. However, the direction of skin sagging is due to the effects of the retaining ligaments' support, not the actual skin descending in the inferomedial direction (Figure 5–54).

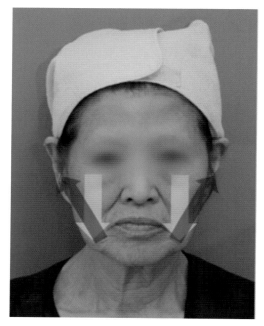

Figure 5–54. Differences between the actual direction of skin sagging and the lifting direction (yellow, direction of gravity; blue, classic lifting direction)

All previous thread lifting and facelift procedures have only described methods of lifting the skin superolaterally, toward the temples or the ears. In fact, this is not precisely opposite the fundamental direction of facial aging. As a result, excessive traction in the superolateral direction to achieve good lifting outcomes leads to unnatural facial expressions and makes the face appear larger. In contrast, gentle traction leads to a reduced lifting effect, so there was previously no other method than to apply a strong lifting effect and persuade the patients even if their face appeared a little larger (Figure 5-55).

We also gave this a lot of thought while continuing to perform the standard techniques and eventually conceived a new lifting method, better suited to the direction of facial aging, by enhancing existing lifting methods. We call this the "vertical lifting technique." With this technique, we aim to correct jowls and nasolabial folds that are difficult to fix with existing superolateral, diagonal lifting techniques. To this end, we lift the jowls, focusing on the anterior malar region, and the skin directly opposite to the direction of gravity, on the basis that facial aging manifests from skin sagging under the influence of gravity. This is also able to alleviate the persistent issues of the cheekbones appearing larger and face appearing wider following conventional lifting procedures.

Vertical lifting requires the use of relatively short threads, 6-9 cm in length, compared to the 17-19-cm threads that are more commonly used. However, with conventionally shaped cog thread, these shorter threads did not have sufficient traction or tensile strength, leading to problems of thread slipping or tissue loosening postoperatively.

Recently, with the development of the molding-type wedge thread, rather than cutting-type cog thread, it has become possible to use short threads with sufficient traction and tensile strength in the procedure.

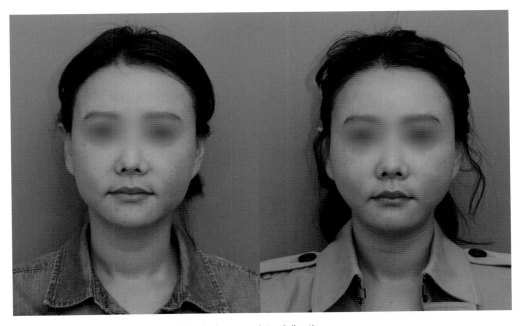

Figure 5-55. Cheekbone and face widening after lifting in the superolateral direction

2. Main clinical indications

The main indications for which the procedure is used clinically are listed below:

1) Desiring gentle lifting

2) Desiring increased anterior malar volume

3) Requiring additional procedures beyond existing methods

4) Severe aging-related skin sagging

5) Prominent cheekbones

3. Instruments

1) 6-9-cm absorbable bidirectional molding wedge thread

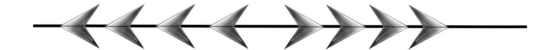

Figure 5–56. Molding–type thread

2) Blunt cannula and anesthetic cannula (liposuction cannula or microcannula used in filler procedures)

3) Dental lidocaine - perioral anesthesia

4) 18-G needle (for entry puncture)

4. Basic design

Three or four 6-9-cm short cog threads are inserted, starting from 1 cm below the lower eyelid; the tips of the cannulae are placed 1 cm above the jawline; and the threads are advanced. Next, the cannulae are removed, the thread is pulled to lift the tissue, and any excess thread is removed.

Subject to circumstances, the space below the cheekbones may be filled, or a modified method can be used to intensively lift only the jowls (Figure 5–57).

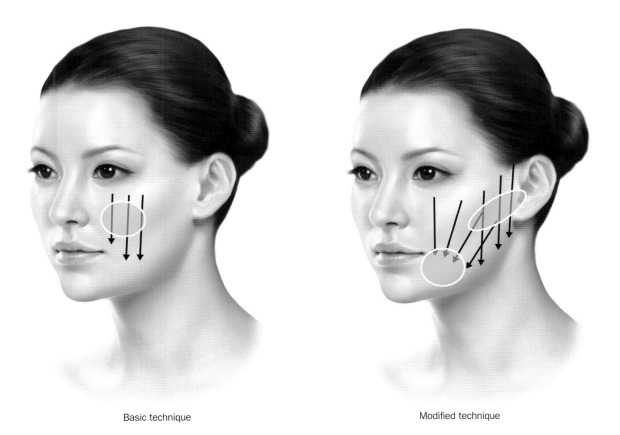

Basic technique

Modified technique

Figure 5–57. Basic design for the vertical lifting technique

5. Surgical procedure

First, infraorbital nerve block is applied. If possible, tumescent fluid should be injected along the designed lines (Figure 5–58).

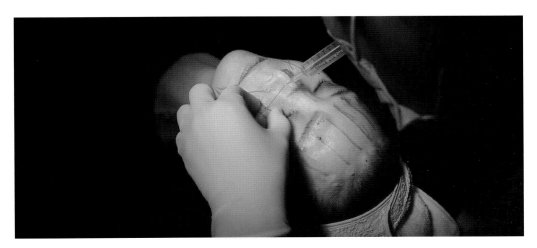

Figure 5–58. Anesthesia

Like common thread lifting procedures, the patient is placed in the extended neck Trendelenburg position, with the upper body tilted slightly posteriorly and the neck extended.

The needles containing the thread are inserted from superior to inferior (Figure 5-59). Three or four threads are inserted from 1cm below the lower eyelid, the tips of the needles are positioned 1cm above the jawline, and the threads are advanced. Here, it is helpful to pinch and raise the tissue of the anterior malar region during insertion.

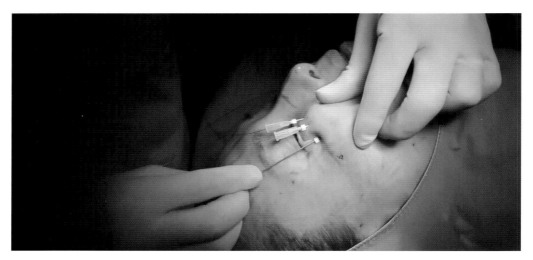

Figure 5-59. Thread insertion

Next, the needles are withdrawn all at once, and the individual threads are pulled to check that they are attached to the tissue (Figures 5-60, 5-61). Here, if any threads come loose, they are removed and re-inserted.

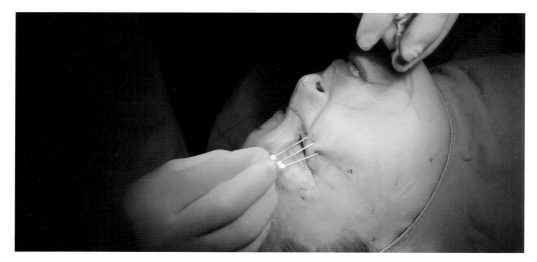

Figure 5-60. Pulling the thread to check the tissue

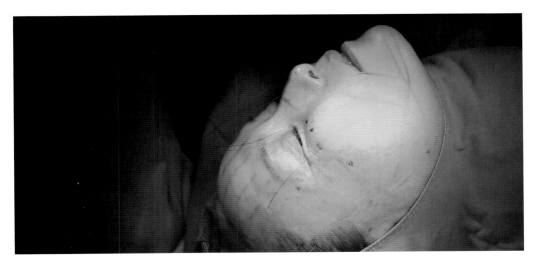

Figure 5-61. Removing the inserted needles

Any excess thread is cut with scissors (Figure 5-62). Here, the skin needs to be pushed slightly during cutting to prevent the thread from re-emerging via the entry site. The area around the entry site is then gently massaged to prevent dimpling.

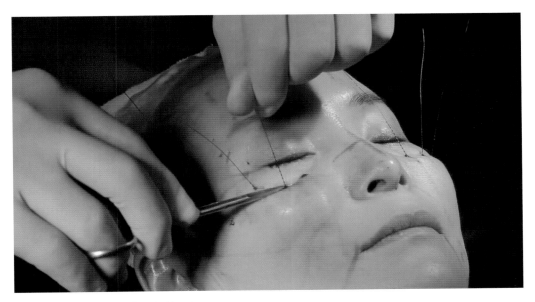

Figure 5-62. Removal of the excess thread with scissors

6. Cautions

The cautions are the same as those for standard thread lifting procedures.

7. Clinical photographs

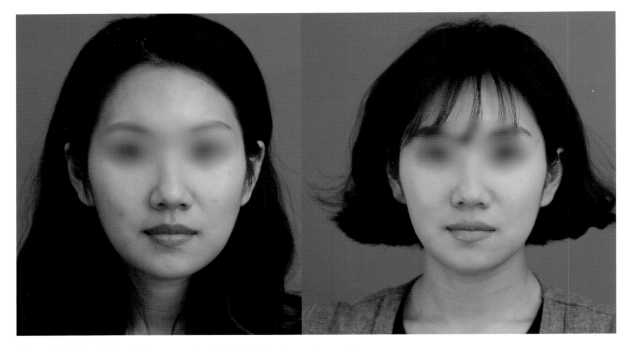

Figure 5-63. Frontal view: (left) preoperative, (right) after 2 postoperative months

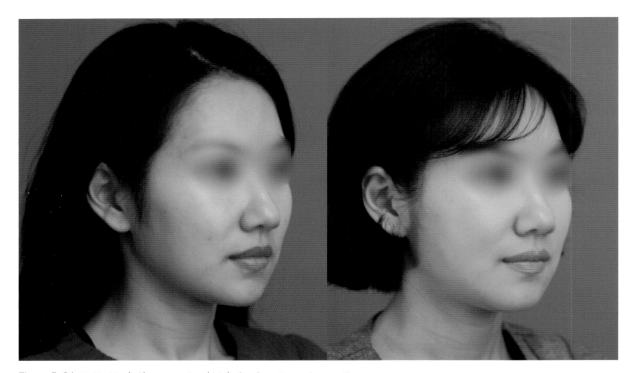

Figure 5-64. Right side: (left) preoperative, (right) after 2 postoperative months

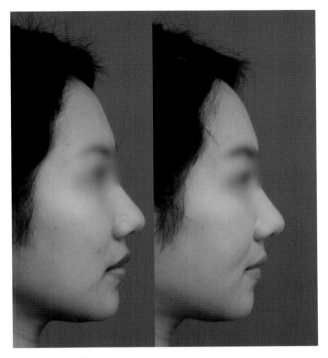

Figure 5-65. Lateral view: (left) preoperative, (right) after 2 postoperative months

[References]

1. Vertical Lifting: A New Optimal Thread Lifting Technique for Asians. Kang SH1, Byun EJ, Kim HS. Dermatol Surg. 2017 Apr 19

TEXTBOOK OF ABSORBABLE THREAD LIFTING

Chapter 06

Case Studies of Surgical Procedures

SECTION 1

Summary of Basic Terms

Currently, there are various shapes and lengths of thread available, so rather than listing the brand names, a summary of terms is required based on the specifications of the thread. In order to avoid confusion about different types of thread, we aim to unify and summarize methods of describing the thread types.

First, cog threads are described according to the thread lengths (the total length and length containing cogs), thread thickness, directionality, cog fabrication method, and width of the cannula or needle used.

Example of specifications

1) Cog thread

Total thread length (cm)	Length of cog section (cm)	Thread thickness	Directionality	Cog fabrication method	Width of cannula or needle
17	9	1–0	Bidirectional	Cutting	18 G (C)
9		–0	Unidirectional	Molding	19 G (N)
44	20	–0	Multidirectional		

For example, 17 (9) cm 1–0 bidirectional cog (cutting) 18 G (C) × 10

Monofilament threads are described according to the total needle length, thread thickness, thread type (mono, multi, twisted), and width of the cannula or needle used.

2) Monofilament thread

Total needle length (cm)	Thread thickness (G)	Thread type	Width of cannula or needle
2.5	28G	Mono	29 G (C)
4	29G	multi	30 G (N)
6	30G	Twisted	31 G (N)
	31G		

For example, 4 cm 6–0 mono 30 G (N) × 50

SECTION 2

Case Studies of Surgical Procedures

Case 01   Soft Jawline and excessive fat below the jaw

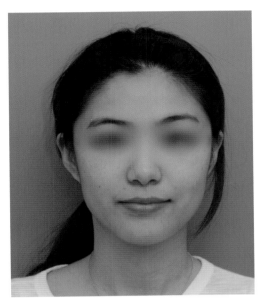
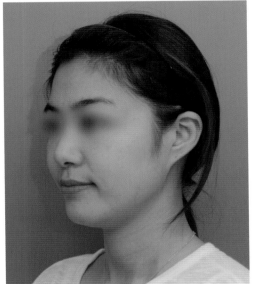

1. Summary

Analysis	1) Skin thickness: thin 2) Cheekbone development: underdeveloped 3) Left–right asymmetry: slight asymmetry 4) Soft jawline 5) Excessive fat below the jaw
Treatment plan	1) Thread lifting, focusing on the lower face and jawline 2) Thread lifting to reduce the fat beneath the jaw
Number and type of threads	1) 17(9) cm 1-0 bidirectional cog (cutting) 18 G (C) × 10 2) 4cm 6-0 mono 30 G (N) × 50
Concomitant treatments	None
Cautions	1) Not to apply excessive lifting force 2) To insert the monofilament thread in the fat layer in the area needing fat reduction
Outcomes	Better defined jawline and loss of fat beneath the jaw

2. Design

Although this patient did not have well-developed cheekbones, because we aimed to correct the jawline, the procedure was performed medially and inferiorly. The thread was placed from behind the ear to below the jaw to correct the area under the jaw.

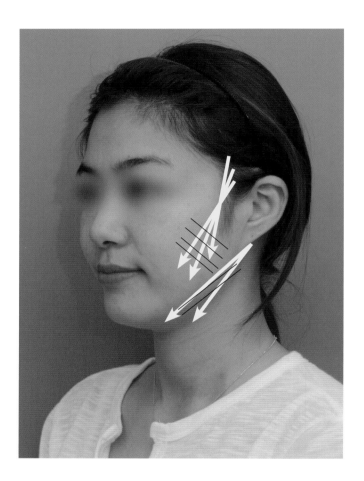

3. Pre- and postoperative photographs

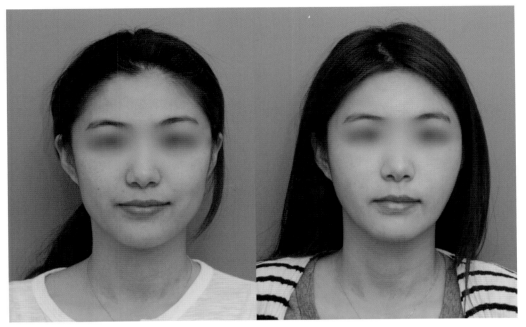

Preoperative frontal view   Postoperative frontal view

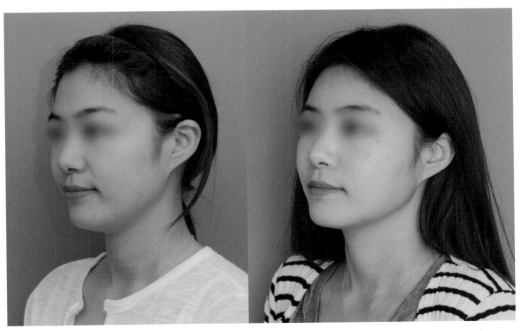

Preoperative lateral view   Postoperative lateral view

Case 02   Soft Jawline and full cheeks

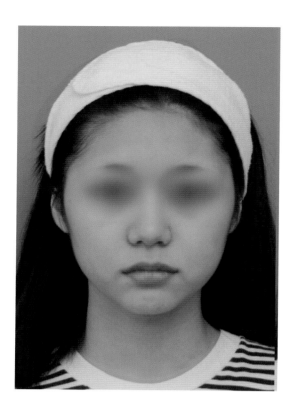

1. Summary

Analysis	1) Skin thickness: average 2) Cheekbone development: small 3) Left–right asymmetry: asymmetric 4) Well–developed bilateral masseter muscles 5) Excessive fat on the jawline and cheeks
Treatment plan	1) Jawline correction rather than lifting 2) Fat reduction on the cheeks and jawline
Number and type of threads	1) 17(9) cm 1-0 bidirectional cog (molding) 18 G (C) × 10 2) 4 cm 6-0 mono 30 G (N) × 50
Concomitant treatments	Masseter muscle reduction using Botox injection
Cautions	1) Not to apply excessive lifting, since the main objective is jawline correction 2) Not to cause bruising when inserting the monofilament thread near the jawline and jowls
Outcomes	1) Follow–up photographs after 3 postoperative months 2) Narrower jaw and loss of fat in the cheeks and jawline

2. Design

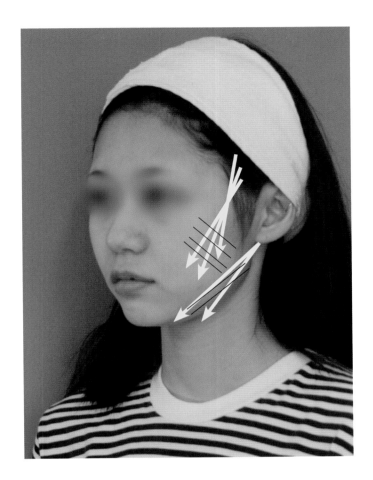

3. Pre- and postoperative photographs

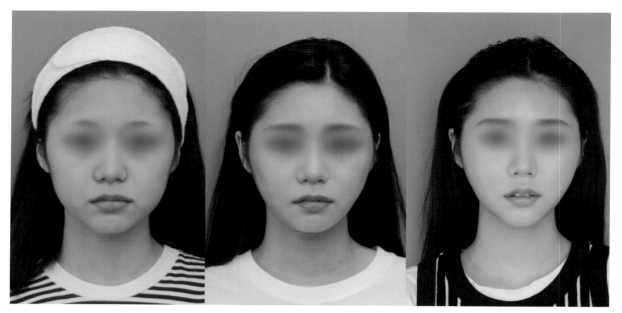

Preoperative   Immediate postoperative   After 2 postoperative months

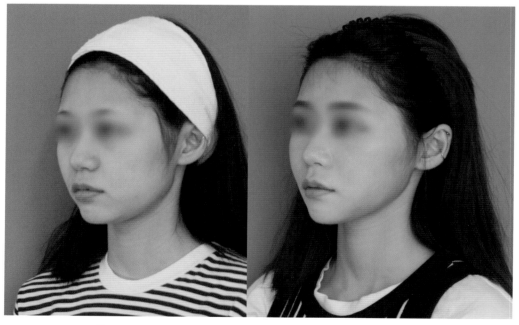

Preoperative   After 2 postoperative months

Case 03   Flat cheeks and downturned oral commissures

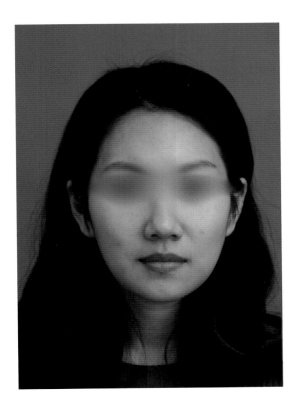

1. Summary

Analysis	1) Skin thickness: average 2) Cheekbone development: small 3) Left–right asymmetry: no asymmetry 4) Flat cheeks 5) Downturned oral commissures
Treatment plan	1) Volume lifting in the anterior malar region 2) Oral commissure lifting
Number and type of threads	1) 9 (6) cm 2-0 bidirectional cog (molding) 21 G (C) × 8 2) 4 cm 6-0 mono 30 G (N) × 30
Concomitant treatments	None
Cautions	1) To accurately mark the location for increasing volume in the anterior malar area preoperatively 2) To gently gather the tissue radially around the jowls 3) To apply a natural lift and loosen the relatively soft skin below the eyes with postoperative massage, since this area can develop dimpling after excessive lifting
Outcomes	Anterior malar volume improvement and oral commissure lifting

2. Design

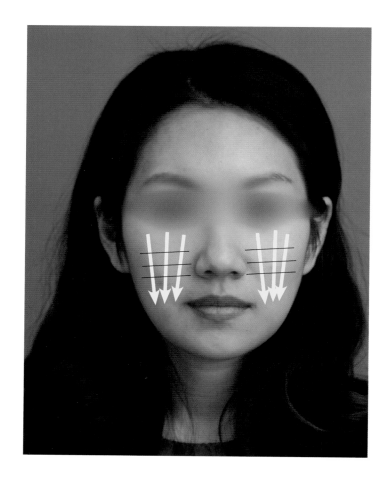

3. Pre- and postoperative photographs

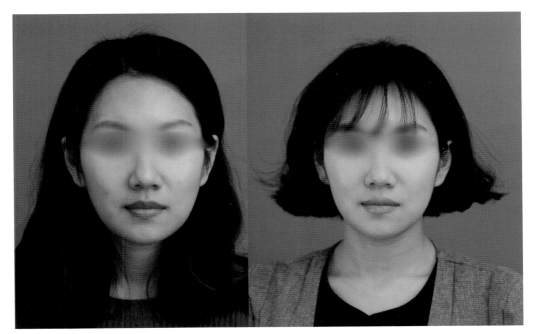

Preoperative   After 2 postoperative months

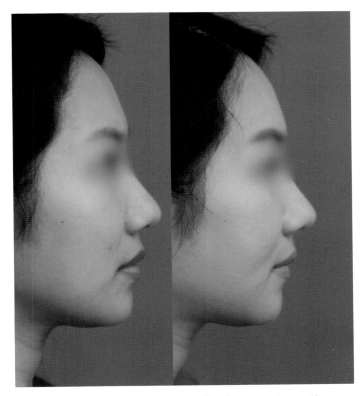

Preoperative   After 2 postoperative months

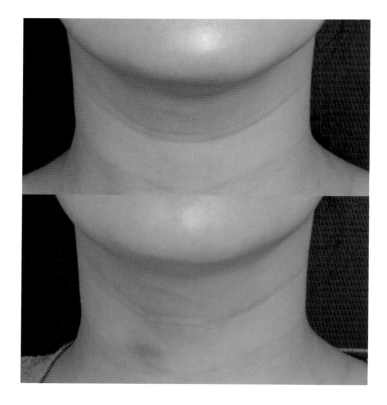

Case 04 Deep neck wrinkles relative to age and sagging fat below

1. Summary

Analysis	1) Skin thickness: thin 2) Cheekbone development: not applicable 3) Left–right asymmetry: not applicable 4) Deep neck wrinkles and fat below the jaw not too severe
Treatment plan	1) Fat reduction below the jaw 2) Neck wrinkle correction

Number and type of threads	1) Fat below the jaw
	   9 (6) cm 2-0 bidirectional cog (molding) 21 G (C) × 10
	   4 cm 6-0 mono 30 G (N) × 40
	2) Neck wrinkles
	   2.5 cm 6–0 mono 21 G (N) × 40

Concomitant treatments	HA filler
Cautions	1) Not to use a long thread due to the sharp angle of the neck and to place the thread at a constant depth 2) To place the thread in the subcutaneous fat layer rather than the dermis layer after fat reduction below the jaw 3) To perform filler therapy after thread lifting
Outcomes	1) Neck wrinkle correction 2) Fat reduction below the jaw

2. Design

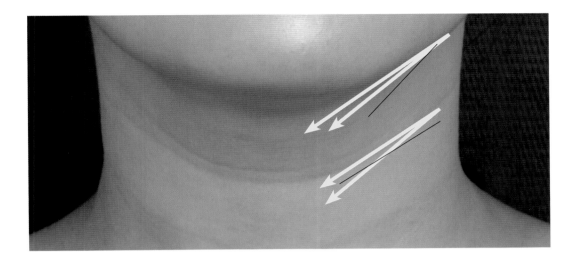

3. Pre- and postoperative photographs

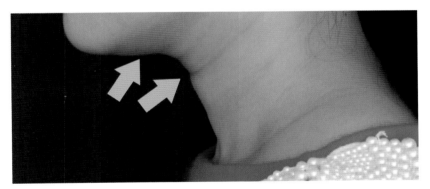

Preoperative

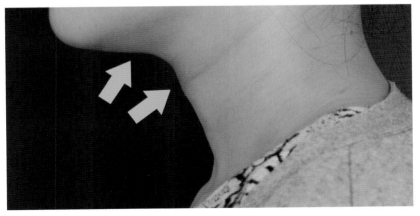

After 2 postoperative months

Case 05   Flat cheeks, sagging cheeks, jowls, and square jawline

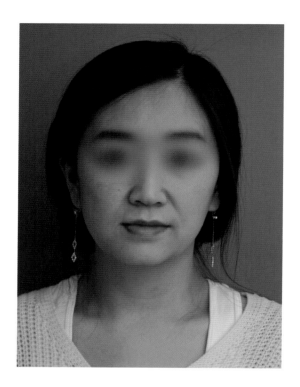

1. Summary

Analysis	1) Skin thickness: average 2) Cheekbone development: small 3) Left–right asymmetry: asymmetric 4) Flat cheeks 5) Downturned oral commissures
Treatment plan	1) Volume improvement in the anterior malar region 2) Oral commissure and jowl improvement
Number and type of threads	1) 9 (6) cm 3–0 multidirectional cog (cutting) 21 G (C) × 8 2) 4 cm 6–0 mono 30 G (N) × 30
Concomitant treatments	None
Cautions	There is a high risk of bleeding and bruising when performing vertical lifting due to the large number of small blood vessels around the orbit. Therefore, care was taken to minimize bleeding and bruising during the operation.
Outcomes	1) Photographs after 3 postoperative weeks Jawline and jowl improvement 2) Bruising was observed on the right cheek immediately after surgery. It took approximately 3 weeks for it to completely resolve.

2. Design

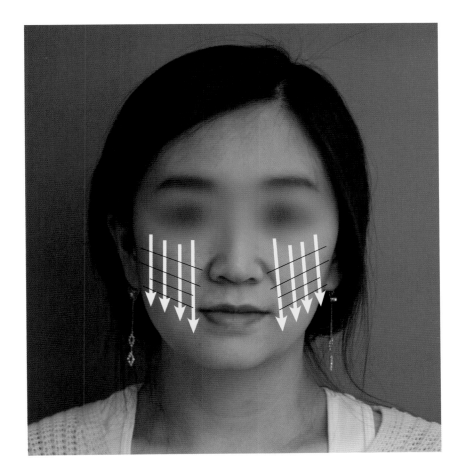

3. Pre- and postoperative photographs

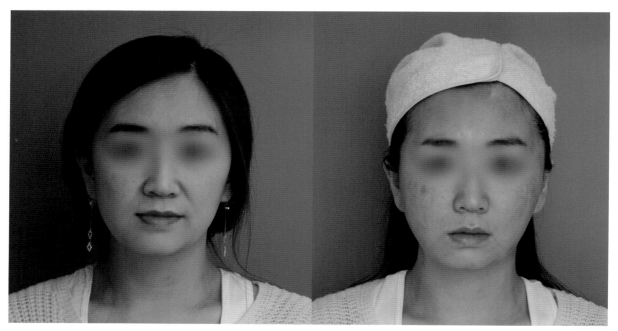

Preoperative   Immediate postoperative

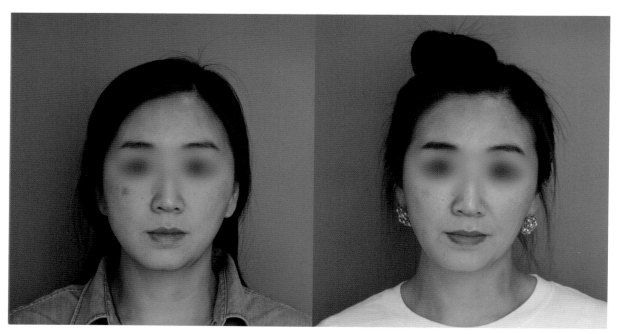

After 1 postoperative week   After 3 postoperative weeks

Case 06 **Sagging eyebrows and shallow forehead wrinkles**

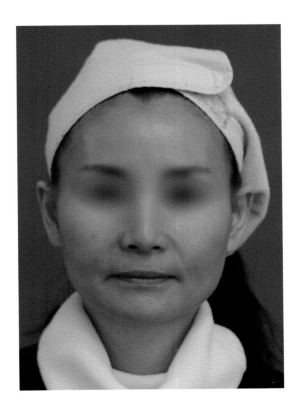

1. Summary

Analysis	1) Skin thickness: average 2) Cheekbone development: not applicable 3) Left–right asymmetry: no asymmetry 4) Slightly sagging eyebrows 5) Loss of elasticity in the skin of the forehead: shallow forehead wrinkles
Treatment plan	1) Correction of shallow forehead wrinkles 2) Forehead lifting
Number and type of threads	1) 9 (6) cm 2-0 bidirectional cog (molding) 21 G (C) × 10 2) 2.5 cm 6-0 mono 30 G (N) × 50
Concomitant treatments	None
Cautions	Since the tissue of the forehead is firmer than other tissues, the lift height is often minimal. For this reason, care was taken not to overreach during the procedure and to lower the patient's expectations of the effects.
Outcomes	1) Photographs after 2 postoperative months 2) Photograph showing approximately 2mm of brow lift

2. Design

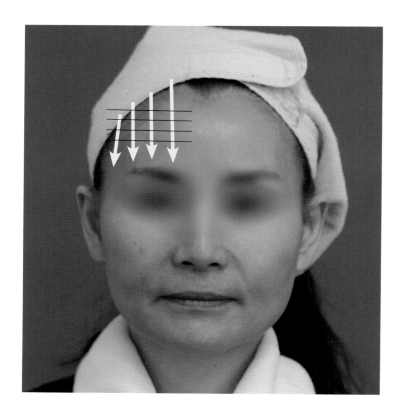

3. Pre- and postoperative photographs

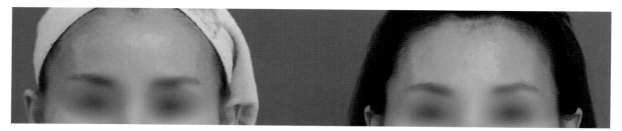

Preoperative

Postoperative

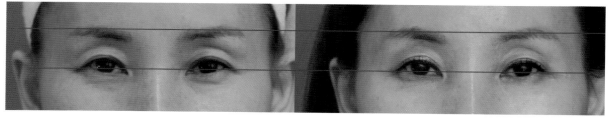

Preoperative

Postoperative

Case 07 Deep, wide wrinkles of the forehead and glabella

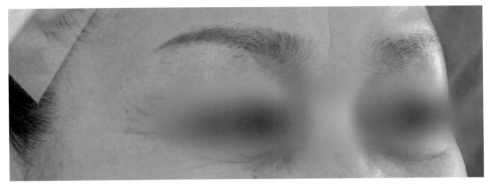

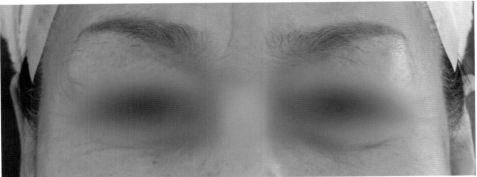

1. Summary

Analysis	1) Skin thickness: thick 2) Cheekbone development: not applicable 3) Left–right asymmetry: no asymmetry 4) Deep wrinkles of the forehead and glabella 　　Clear wrinkles even with a still face 　　Difficult to correct with filler or Botox therapy
Treatment plan	Inserting threads below the deep wrinkles of the forehead and glabella in order to lift the tissue
Number and type of threads	1) 6(3) cm 1-0 multidirectional cog (cutting) 21 G (C) × 20 2) 2.5 cm 6-0 mono 30 G (N) × 30
Concomitant treatments	Forehead and glabellar Botox injection
Cautions	1) The deep wrinkles of the forehead and glabella cannot be easily corrected with filler therapy. In particular, the risk of vascular obstruction in the glabella makes aggressive filler therapy difficult. 2) In such cases, thread lifting can be a good choice. 3) Care was taken not to place the thread too shallow. 4) The appropriate number of threads to insert is 2 – 3 threads per wrinkle. 5) Although the wrinkles themselves do not disappear after treatment, they can show greater improvement compared with that in filler injection.
Outcomes	Photographs after 1 postoperative month

2. Design

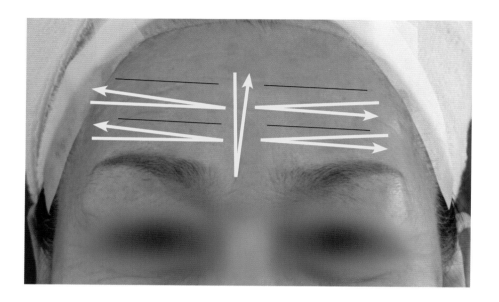

3. Pre- and postoperative photographs

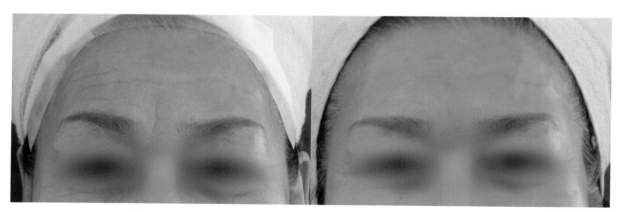

Preoperative

Postoperative

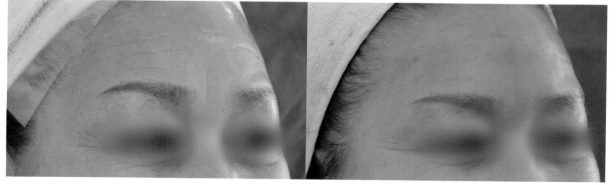

After 1 postoperative month

After 1 postoperative month

Case 08　Sagging cheeks, deep nasolabial folds, and jowls

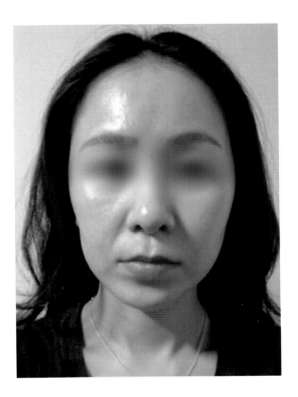

1. Summary

Analysis	1) Skin thickness: thin 2) Cheekbone development: underdeveloped 3) Left–right asymmetry: asymmetric 4) Narrow face 5) Did not want the cheekbones to appear larger 6) Worried about downtime and swelling immediately after the procedure
Treatment plan	1) Operating on the area below the cheekbones 2) Nasolabial fold and jowl correction 3) Overall enhancement of skin elasticity 4) Minimizing swelling 5) Using a tie technique
Number and type of threads	1) 7(7) cm 1-0 unidirectional cog (cutting) 18 G (C) × 8 2) 4 cm 6-0 mono 30 G (N) × 50
Concomitant treatments	None
Cautions	1) This case had a high likelihood of a positive postoperative outcome. 2) Care was taken not to apply excessive traction in lifting. 3) We made sure to insert the knot securely beneath the skin.
Outcomes	1) Photographs after 1 postoperative month 2) Correction of nasolabial folds and jowls

2. Design

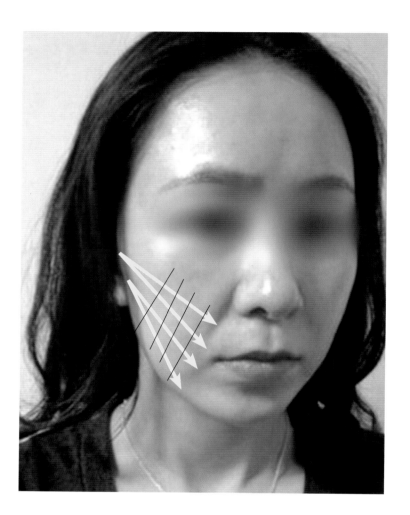

3. Pre- and postoperative photographs

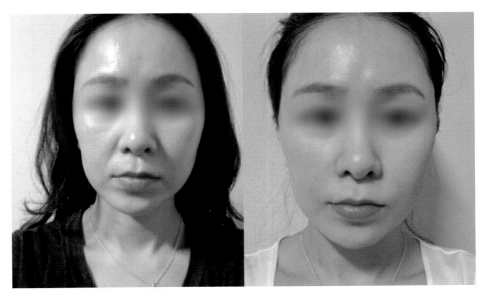

Preoperative frontal view   Postoperative frontal view

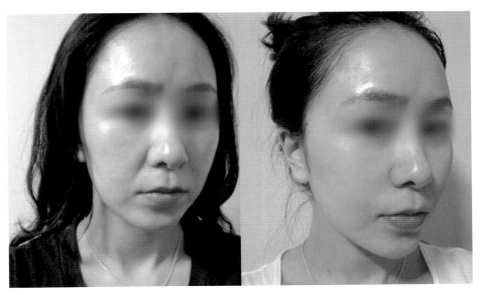

Preoperative side view   Postoperative side view

Case 09 Nasolabial folds, marionette lines, jowls, cheekbones, forehead, and temples

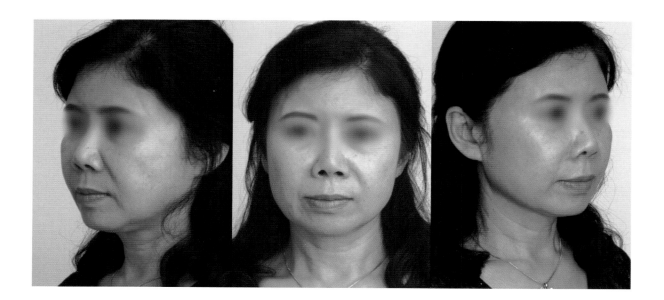

1. Summary

Analysis	1) Skin thickness: thick 2) Cheekbone development: large 3) Left–right asymmetry: asymmetric 4) Typical facial structure of East Asian women 5) Full cheeks 6) Prominent nasolabial folds and jowls
Treatment plan	1) Fat graft 　Increasing volume in the forehead, temples, and below the eyes 2) Thread lifting 　Avoid making the cheekbones larger 　Combining with vertical lifting 　Due to the large number of threads being used, the overall tension needs to be carefully managed. The procedure is performed without excessive anchoring.
Number and type of threads	1) 17(9) cm 1-0 bidirectional cog (molding) 18 G (C) × 10 2) 9(6) cm 2-0 bidirectional cog (molding) 21 G (C) × 4 3) 4 cm 6-0 mono 30 G (N) × 50
Concomitant treatments	Fat graft (forehead, temples, and below the eyes)
Cautions	1) In order to maintain the facial symmetry, thread lifting was combined with fat graft in the forehead, temples, nasolabial area, and below the eyes. 2) This patient had large cheekbones and somewhat firm skin, so in order to maximize the lifting effect, there is a tendency to apply a strong lift. This would cause the cheekbones to appear more prominent, such that, even if the lift effect is good, the face can appear larger, reducing patient satisfaction. 3) We aimed to improve the patient's appearance through overall symmetry.
Outcomes	1) Photographs after 2 postoperative months 2) Overall softer face 3) Correction of sagging without making the face appear large

2. Design

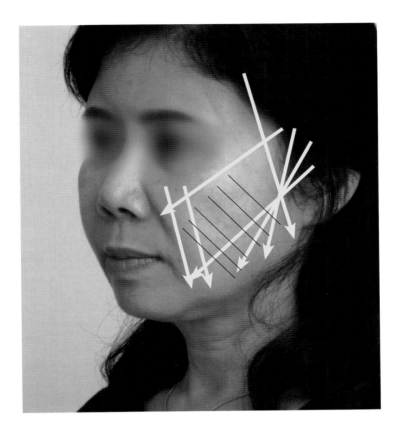

3. Pre- and postoperative photographs

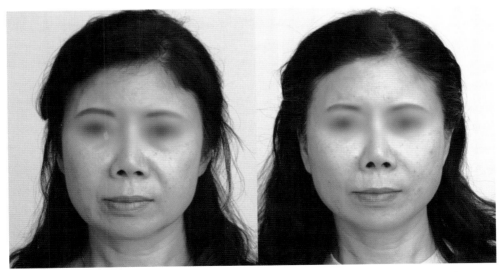

Preoperative   Frontal view after 2 postoperative months

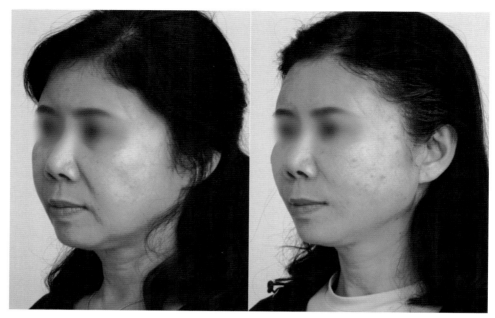

Preoperative   Lateral view after 2 postoperative months

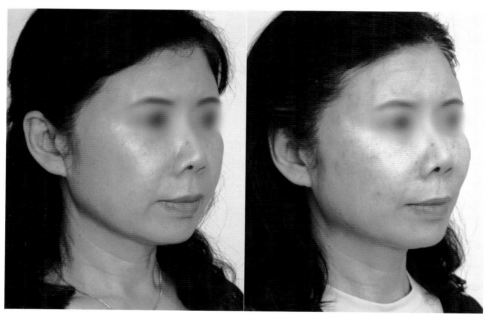

Preoperative   Lateral view after 2 postoperative months

Case 10   Marionette lines, jowls, nasolabial folds, cheekbones, and sagging of the lower face

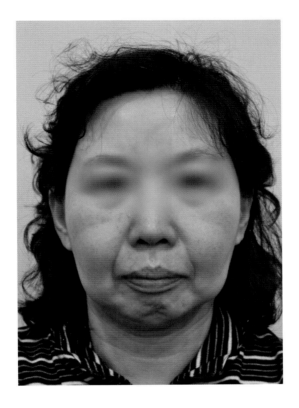

1. Summary

Analysis	1) Skin thickness: thick 2) Cheekbone development: large 3) Left–right asymmetry: relatively less asymmetry 4) Typical facial structure of East Asian women 5) Full cheeks 6) Prominent nasolabial folds and jowls
Treatment plan	1) Although this patient was a candidate for facelift surgery, she wanted thread lifting, so we had to use an anchoring–type method. 2) Due to the patient's thick skin, it was absolutely necessary to use an anchoring–type method. 3) Particular care was taken not to make the cheekbones larger.
Number and type of threads	45 cm 3-0 unidirectional cog (cutting) 18 G (C) with Loop: V-Loc thread × 8
Concomitant treatments	None
Cautions	1) This patient required facelift surgery due to her large cheekbones, thick and firm skin, and severe sagging. For this reason, it was necessary to use an anchoring–type technique to provide a powerful lifting effect. 2) This patient had large cheekbones, so if an anchoring–type technique is used to correct the nasolabial folds, it could easily cause the cheekbones to appear more prominent, such that, even if the lift effect is good, the face can appear larger, reducing patient satisfaction. 3) We paid close attention to this possibility while correcting sagging of the lower face. 4) In cases like this, fat graft or filler injection can help improve the nasolabial folds.
Outcomes	1) Photographs after 1 postoperative month 2) The lower face was lifted overall, and the patient appeared younger with a softer face. 3) Even though this patient required facelift surgery, we were able to correct sagging of the face using an anchoring–type technique, without making the face appear wider.

2. Design

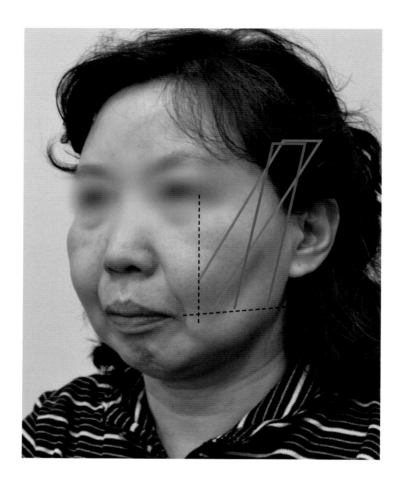

3. Pre- and postoperative photographs

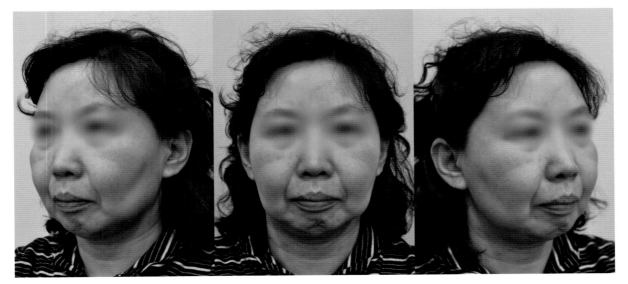

Preoperative

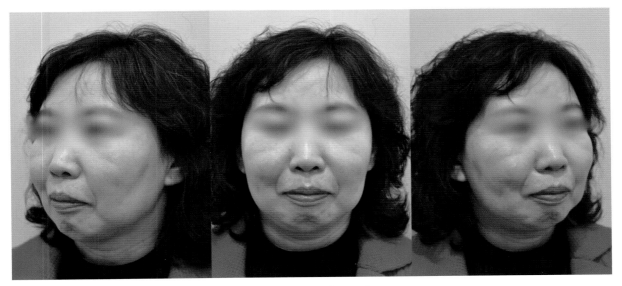

After 1 postoperative month

Case 11   Jowls, square jaw, marionette lines, nasolabial folds, and sagging of the lower face

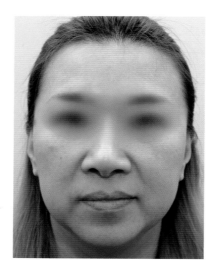

1. Summary

Analysis	1) Skin thickness: thick 2) Cheekbone development: moderate 3) Left–right asymmetry: somewhat asymmetric 4) Full cheeks 5) Prominent nasolabial folds and jowls 6) Prominent mid–cheek furrows
Treatment plan	1) Due to the patient's thick skin, an anchoring–type technique had to be considered, but the patient did not want this, having experienced severe temporal pain following an anchoring–type procedure using non–absorbable suture thread 10 years previously. 2) For this reason, we decided on using a floating–type technique using absorbable suture thread. 3) Vertical lifting using short threads was considered to correct the mid–cheek furrows. 4) Though the patient does not have especially large cheekbones, she did not want her face to become wider, so filler injections were administered to correct the nasolabial folds.
Number and type of threads	1) 17(9) cm 1-0 bidirectional cog (molding) 12 G (C) × 12 2) 9(6) cm 1-0 bidirectional cog (molding) 18 G (C) × 8
Concomitant treatments	Filler injections – to correct the nasolabial folds, hyaluronic acid filler was administered, with 1mL in each side.
Cautions	1) This patient could have been considered for facelift surgery given her thick skin and large amount of sagging, relative to her age. Therefore, an anchoring–type technique requiring strong traction would have been appropriate. However, the patient did not want an anchoring–type technique, having experienced temporal pain as a side effect of a previous anchoring–type procedure. 2) Recently, floating–type methods with a molding–type thread are also showing positive outcomes, so we determined that a sufficiently good outcome could be achieved even with a floating–type technique. 3) If the effect of thread lifting is predicted to be somewhat insufficient, filler or fat injection is recommended in the areas of the mid–cheek furrows, nasolabial folds, and marionette lines.
Outcomes	1) Photographs after 6 postoperative months 2) Overall lifting of the lower face, resulting in a narrower face 3) Although this was a patient who required facelift surgery, correction of face sagging has been maintained for 6 months using a floating–type technique. 4) As described above, additional filler or fat injections are thought to be required for the nasolabial folds, mid–cheek furrows, and marionette lines. 5) Most importantly, if this level of lifting effect can be achieved without symptoms such as temporal pain, the patient is willing to receive regular treatments.

2. Design

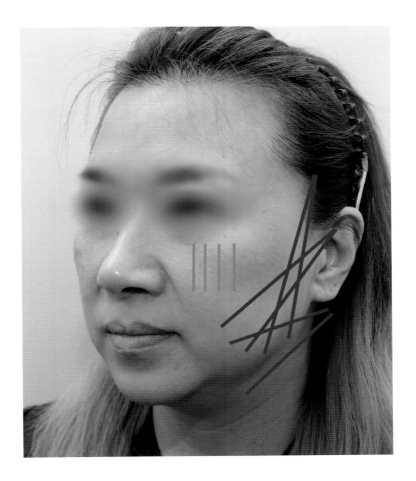

3. Pre- and postoperative photographs

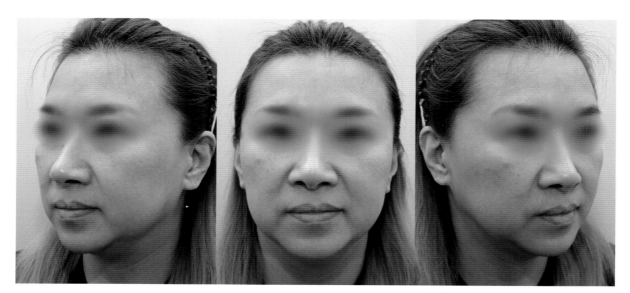

Preoperative

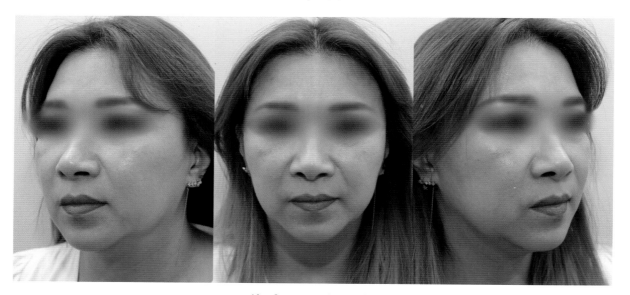

After 6 postoperative months

Case 12　Marionette lines, jowls, and square jaw

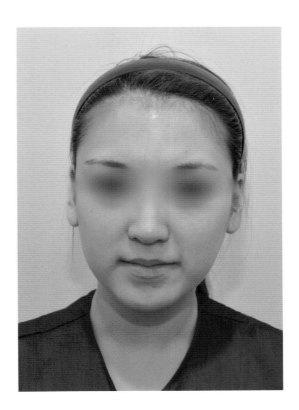

1. Summary

Analysis	1) Skin thickness: average 2) Cheekbone development: moderate 3) Left–right asymmetry: moderate asymmetry 4) Moderate sagging of the cheeks
Treatment plan	1) An anchoring–type technique with strong traction was considered since the patient wanted a narrower jawline. 2) Fat injection was considered to improve the patient's flat forehead and provide volume.
Number and type of threads	45cm 3–0 unidirectional cog (cutting) 18 G (C) with Loop: V–Loc thread × 8
Concomitant treatments	Fat injection – flat forehead correction
Cautions	1) Although the patient had moderately sized cheekbones, if an anchoring–type technique alone was used to correct the nasolabial folds, the cheekbones would be widened, and the patient's face could appear larger. 2) Therefore, we focused on generating skin traction in the vertical direction in order to improve sagging.
Outcomes	1) Photographs after 1 postoperative month 2) The lower face was lifted in a vertical direction, giving the face a narrower outline. 3) The marionette lines were also improved.

2. Design

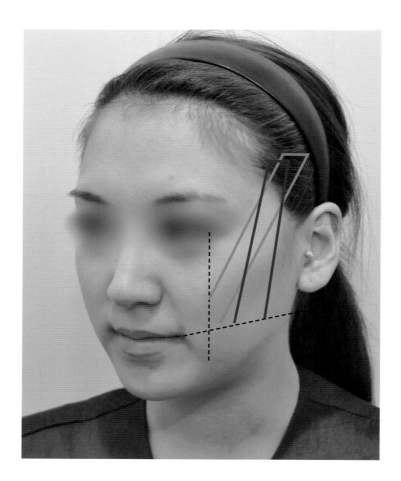

3. Pre- and postoperative photographs

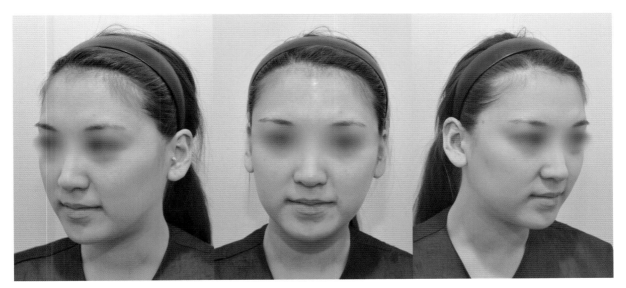

Preoperative

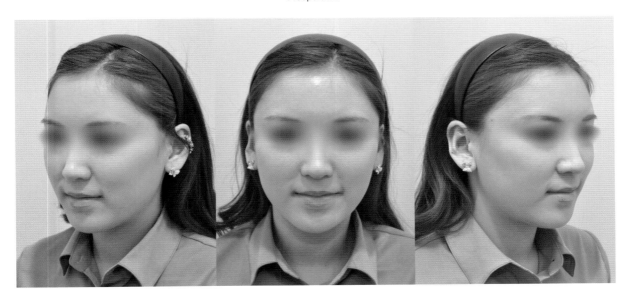

After 1 postoperative month

Case 13   Broad jawline

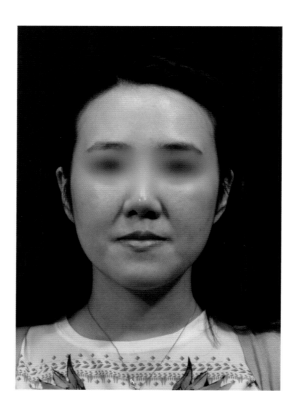

1. Summary

Analysis	1) Skin thickness: somewhat thick 2) Cheekbone development: underdeveloped 3) Left–right asymmetry: not too severe 4) Relatively broad jawline
Treatment plan	1) Lifting to make a narrower jawline (V–line) 2) The skin did not show much movement when pulled manually; therefore, in order to maximize the effect of the treatment, we decided to perform anchoring–type thread lifting.
Number and type of threads	44(20) cm 1-0 bidirectional cog (molding) 17 G (C) × 4 17(10) cm 1-0 multidirectional cog (molding) 18 G (C) × 8
Concomitant treatments	None
Cautions	1) Since pulling strongly on the area directly next to the oral commissure is likely to result in dimpling, this area should be approached conservatively. 2) In order to prevent excessive dimpling, it is helpful to insert the multidirectional cog thread directly next to the bidirectional thread to suppress excessive contraction.
Outcomes	Narrower jawline

2. Design

1) In order to induce strong lifting at the jawline, we marked two points on the scalp over the temporal fascia and inserted the thread according to the pattern shown in the figure below.

2) Two entry sites for the thread were marked on the right and left side of the hairline, at a height approximately 1.5 cm above the superior margin of the eyebrows.

3) Lines were drawn vertically inferior from the lateral canthus and oral commissure to the mandibular angle. Points were marked at the intersection of these two lines and at 1-cm intervals along the horizontal line to indicate the exit sites for the thread (four exit sites on each side of the face).

4) In order to prevent skin dimpling due to excessive contraction, a multidirectional cog thread was inserted immediately next to the line connecting the scalp to the jawline.

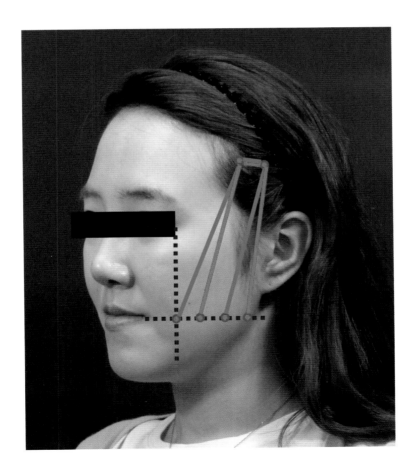

3. Pre- and postoperative photographs

1) After 3 postoperative days

The jawline appears narrower, but there is still some swelling around the cheekbones.

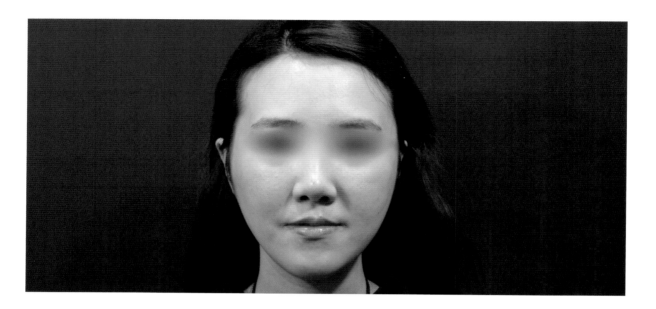

2) After 2 postoperative weeks

The swelling around the cheekbones has subsided, and the patient's face appears more natural.

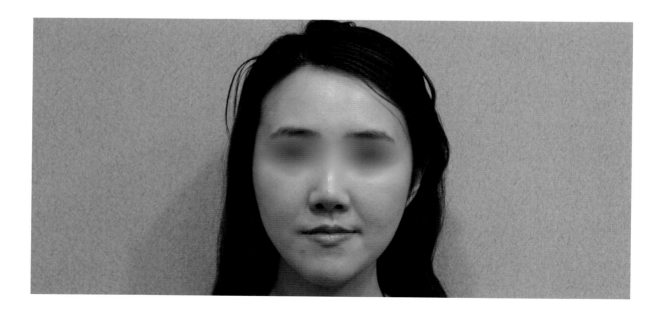

Case 14   Nasolabial folds and marionette lines

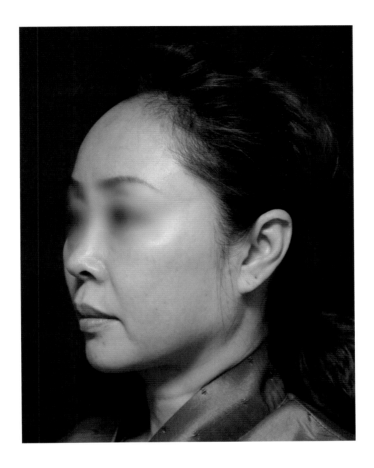

1. Summary

Analysis	1) Skin thickness: somewhat thin 2) Cheekbone development: somewhat developed
Treatment plan	Since the patient expected a strong effect, we decided to perform anchoring–type thread lifting.
Number and type of threads	44(20) cm 1-0 bidirectional cog (molding) 17 G (C) × 4 17(10) cm 1-0 multidirectional cog (molding) 18 G (C) × 8
Concomitant treatments	None
Cautions	When strong lifting is performed in patients with thin skin and hollow cheeks, the cheeks can show a collapsed appearance. Therefore, it is important to provide lifting with appropriate strength. If necessary, before the consultation, the patient should be informed about volume correction treatments such as fat grafting or filler injection.
Outcomes	1) After 1 postoperative month, the patient showed considerable improvements in the nasolabial folds and marionette lines. 2) The jawline, especially near the mandibular angle, had become narrower.

2. Design

1) Two entry sites for the thread were marked on the right and left side of the hairline, at a height approximately 1.5 cm above the superior margin of the eyebrows.

2) Lines were drawn vertically inferior from the lateral canthus and oral commissure to the mandibular angle. Points were marked at the intersection of these two lines and at 1-cm intervals along the horizontal line to indicate the exit sites for the thread (four exit sites on each side of the face).

3) In order to prevent skin dimpling due to excessive contraction, a multidirectional cog thread was inserted immediately next to the line connecting the scalp to the jawline.

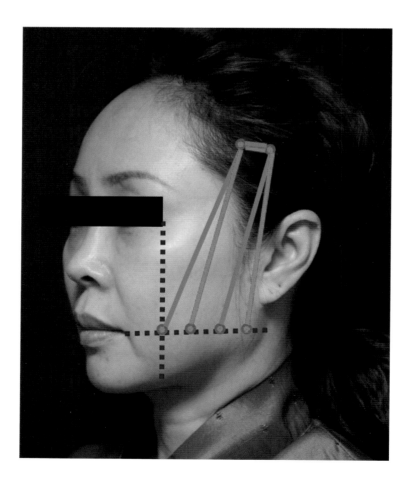

3. Pre- and postoperative photographs

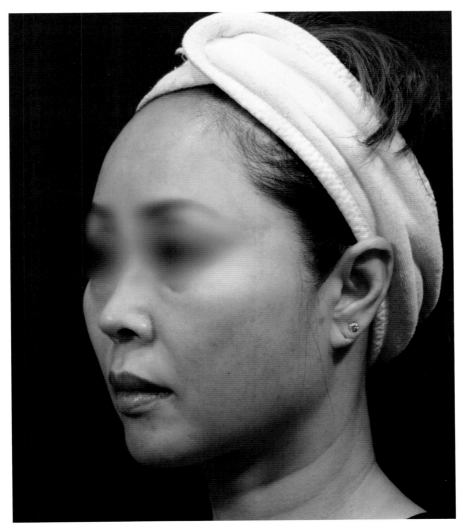

After 1 postoperative month

TEXTBOOK OF ABSORBABLE THREAD LIFTING

Chapter

07

Postoperative Management

SECTION 1

Immediately after Surgery

1) In order to minimize postoperative swelling, ice should be applied on the cheek area for the first 3 days, and pillows should be used to elevate the upper body during sleep.

2) On the day of surgery, patients should not wash their face in the evening but simply apply the lotion provided by the hospital before sleeping. They should be instructed to wash their face the next morning.

3) If there is any skin dimpling after surgery, this should be immediately relieved by massage. If this persists for more than 4 weeks, fibrosis may occur, resulting in permanent dimpling. Therefore, it is important to observe the patient's course carefully during this period and treat any skin dimpling.

4) Although bruising is not common, it can develop sometimes. In this case, it should naturally subside within 1-2 weeks. A bruise cream can be used to aid this process.

5) In some cases, patients cannot close their eyes, or the corners of their mouths move up and down immediately after the surgery; this is due to the effects of anesthesia and should improve after a day. The patient should be informed of this possibility before the procedure and reassured if any such symptoms arise. In the case of symptoms, the patient must be examined directly.

SECTION 2

Prescription Examples

For patients undergoing general lifting procedures, we recommend prescribing antibiotics. We usually issue a prescription for 3 days. Below, we present an sample prescription of an antibiotic, anti-inflammatory analgesic, and gastroprotective agent (Table 7-1).

Table 7-1. Sample prescription

Cecrocin capsule®	tid
Afentac®	tid
Newbis®	tid

In the case of anchoring-type techniques, due to temporal pain, we additionally issue a 7-day prescription for an analgesic, antacid, and sleeping pill (Table 7-2).

Table 7-2. Sample prescription after anchoring-type thread lifting

Cecrocin capsule®	tid
Radine tablet®	75 mg bid
Clanza tablet®	bid
Tylenol ER®	tid
Solondo®	5 mg bid
Xanax®	0.25 mg gdhs

SECTION 3

Home Care

1) As far as possible, the patient should rest and avoid excessive exercise or movement.

2) In terms of food, we recommend a soft, liquid diet; if the patient wants to eat a normal diet, they should avoid tough or chewy foods.

3) In order to minimize postoperative swelling, ice should be applied on the patient's cheeks for the first 3 days, and pillows should be used to elevate the upper body during sleep.

4) On the day of surgery, patients should not wash their face in the evening, and only apply the lotion provided by the hospital before sleeping. They should be instructed to wash their face the next morning.

SECTION 4

Cautions

1) In particular, the patient should be careful in yawning or otherwise opening their mouth widely and avoid hard foods or tough meat for around 4 weeks.

2) The patient should be warned not to touch or rub the treated area.

3) The patient can begin gentle exercise after 3-4 postoperative days, but we recommend avoiding vigorous exercise such as massages, jogging, or the gym for 3-4 weeks.

4) Hair treatments, such as perming or dying, are allowed after one month.

5) The patient should avoid overly hot environments such as the sauna, drinking alcohol, and intense exercise for one week. This is because swelling can become more severe when exposed to heat.

6) The needle marks in the treated area usually fade after 2-3 days.

7) Although the face will show postoperative swelling on the day of the operation, most of the swelling subsides within 2-3 days. If the thread has been anchored to the scalp, there may be some swelling above the cheekbones and in the temporal area; this usually subsides after about one week.

8) Usually, when a barbed thread has been used, the patient may experience burning pain when the area posterior to thread insertion is touched or irritated. This feeling typically disappears within 1-2 weeks.

9) Rarely, skin dimpling can occur near the end of the inserted thread after 2 weeks to one month. In such cases, it is essential for the patient to visit the hospital and have the dimpling treated by massage.

10) In patients who frequently use their facial muscles, skin dimpling can occur even after one month has passed. This is due to the ends of the thread catching on the skin after excessive skin movement and can be resolved by massaging the affected area.

11) Even after one month has passed, a sudden popping noise may be heard in the area of thread lifting when the patient chews food or smiles broadly. Since this will not cause a reduction in the lifting effect, concerned patients should be thoroughly reassured.

TEXTBOOK OF ABSORBABLE
THREAD LIFTING

Chapter 08

Adverse Effects, Prevention, and Treatment

Although various undesired effects occur after thread lifting, there are relatively few severe adverse effects. Most of these adverse effects are transient and resolve spontaneously, so thread lifting can be performed without much concern. Here, we list the most commonly observed adverse effects in our clinical experience and briefly discuss means for prevention and treatment.

SECTION 1

Facial asymmetry

Facial asymmetry commonly develops immediately after surgery. Asymmetry due to excessive traction on one side should be corrected by massage. However, asymmetry is usually caused by swelling differences, which can persist for 1-2 weeks but will spontaneously resolve over time.

Asymmetry needs to be corrected if it persists beyond 3-4 weeks. In addition, most people show some differences between the two sides of their face, but when asymmetry becomes apparent after treatment, they tend to believe that the asymmetry was caused by the treatment. Therefore, it is important to leave a record of preoperative clinical photographs and explain about asymmetry to the patient in advance.

SECTION 2

Ecchymosis and Hematoma

Since thread lifting often uses needles, it is difficult to perform the procedure without any bruising. However, severe bruising requires long recovery times, which is a burden on both the surgeon and patient. For this reason, it is important to minimize bruising as far as possible.

Surgeons should be aware that if bruising develops in the temporal area, the bruise can descend inferiorly or toward the eyes.

The risk of bruising can be reduced considerably by using a cannula instead of a needle or applying anesthesia with an injection containing a vasoconstrictor such as epinephrine. In this case, we recommend waiting for at least 5 min after the anesthetic injection before beginning the procedure.

Hematomas are rare, but in order to prevent hematoma formation, if there is any bleeding during the procedure, the procedure should be stopped, and pressure should be applied at the

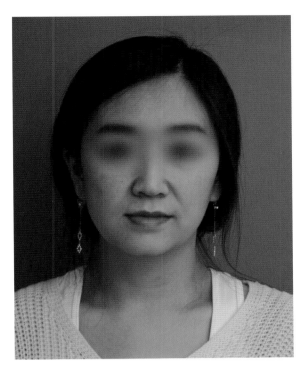

Figure 8-1. Preoperative

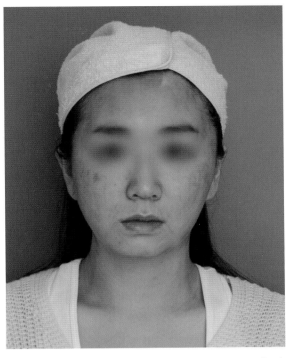

Figure 8-2. Photograph of bruising below the eye immediately after surgery

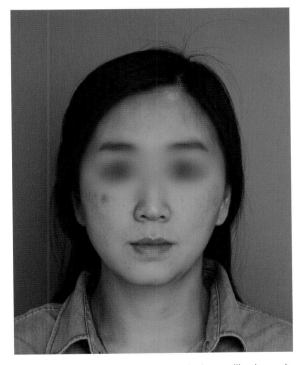

Figure 8-3. After 1 postoperative week, the swelling has subsided but bruising is still visible

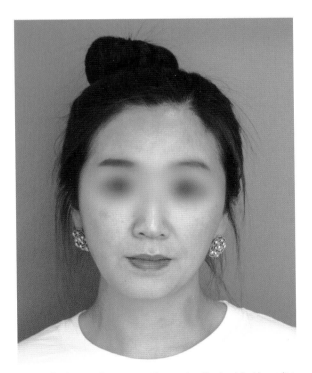

Figure 8-4. After 3 postoperative weeks, the bruising is no longer visible

site of bleeding for 5 min, continuing with the procedure once hemostasis has been confirmed. Severe hematomas need to be removed surgically, but most hematomas can be treated without inflammation by administering antibiotics.

SECTION 3

Pain

After thread lifting, some patients experience foreign body sensation when moving their face, especially when making facial expressions, speaking, or eating. Barbed thread causes more irritation to the surrounding tissue than non-barbed thread and is more likely to cause pain. The experience of pain is different for every patient, ranging from a slight foreign body sensation to difficulty sleeping due to pain. Generally, pain is more severe in those with thicker rather than thinner thread and barbed thread rather than non-barbed thread. In terms of surgical techniques, anchorage in the deep fascia is associated with more severe pain.

In particular, movements of the facial muscles during changes of facial expression and movements of the masseter muscle during chewing can cause severe pain when there is irritation. Therefore, the patient should be careful not to make excessive facial expressions or consume hard or tough foods. During sleeping, pressure near the site of thread insertion can also cause severe pain, so patients are advised to sleep on their backs for at least one week.

Although pain can subside after as few as 1-2 days, patients usually complain of discomfort for about 2 weeks and occasionally experience pain for several months. However, in absorbable thread lifting, because the thread is absorbed, the pain normally resolves spontaneously. Some patients complain of headaches within 2 postoperative weeks. In cases of pain accompanied by swelling, surgeons should be aware of the possibilities of hematoma or infection.

SECTION 4

Palpable Thread

When using thicker thread, if the thread is placed close to the surface and the patient has thin skin, the thread may be palpable beneath the skin. When using absorbable thread, this normally resolves naturally, but when the patient experiences significant discomfort or there is a risk of scarring, the thread should be aggressively removed. In particular, in patients with thin skin, it is important to use a thin thread and insert it at a deep level, if possible.

If the end of the thread is palpable, after making a 1.5-2-mm incision, pressing the skin over the palpable thread end should cause the thread to protrude out of the skin, allowing it to be removed; if this is unsuccessful, the thread can be removed using narrow mosquito forceps. If the center of the thread is palpable, after making a 1.5-2-mm incision, the thread can be removed using small forceps or a skin hook.

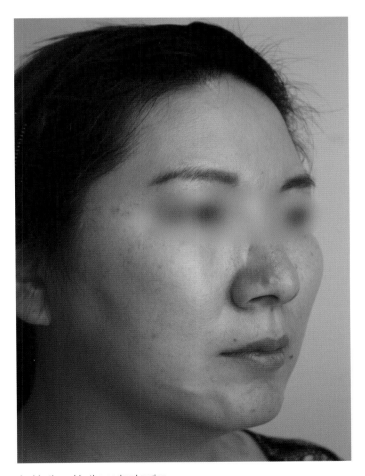

Figure 8-5. A case of visible, palpable thread in the perioral region

SECTION 5

Skin Dimples

Skin dimpling refers to concavity of the inferior skin like a dimple (Figure 8-6). Sometimes, postoperative skin dimples are deliberately left in an effort to induce a stronger lifting effect and can also occur later, after 1-2 postoperative weeks. Severe skin dimples should be actively resolved as soon as possible; if they persist for more than 1 month, it can lead to adhesion, making them difficult to eliminate, so it is best to resolve any dimples within one postoperative month. Most dimples disappear with firm massaging in the opposite direction to the barbs within 3-4 postoperative weeks. Since this treatment can cause pain, we recommend administering a local anesthetic injection.

If massage does not fix the dimpling, the thread should be removed. Since the patient is sometimes unaware of dimpling, it is crucial to perform follow-up monitoring within 4 postoperative weeks.

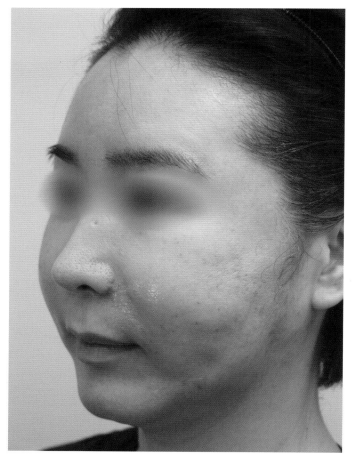

Figure 8-6. Postoperative skin dimpling

SECTION 6

Worsening of Mid-cheek Furrows

In patients with well-defined mid-cheek furrow, the mid-cheek furrows can actually become worse after thread lifting. It is important to check the state of the mid-cheek furrows before thread lifting (Figure 8-7).

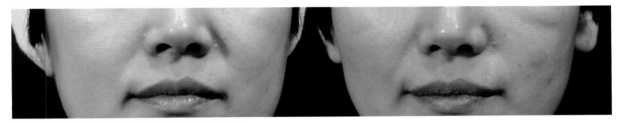

Figure 8-7. Worsening of the tear troughs

SECTION 7

Thread Migration and Protrusion

When using a cog thread, the thread can migrate upward or downward and protrude like a pimple (Figures 8-8, 8-9). This occurs when the anchor point is too weak and the thread cannot resist the forces pulling in the opposite direction. When using bidirectional barbed thread, it is important to avoid damage to the barbs. As far as possible, the thread should be inserted such that there is a similar length of thread with barbs facing in each direction. If the end of the thread is pushing out the skin like a pimple, the skin should be penetrated using an 18-G needle and microforceps or a similar instrument used to pull out the thread. If the thread needs to be removed, it is important not to cut part of the thread but rather to remove the whole thread. If the thread is already protruding out from the skin, the thread can be removed by pulling. It is important to understand that the location of thread protrusion is often unrelated to the original direction of the thread.

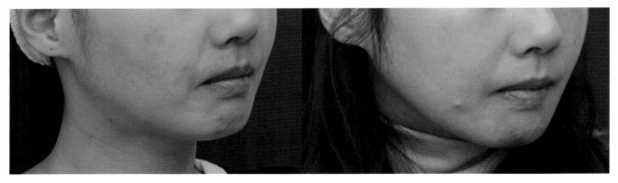

Figure 8-8. Postoperative thread protrusion A

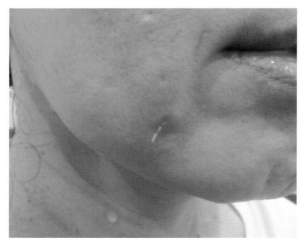

Figure 8-9. Postoperative thread protrusion B

SECTION 8

Infection

The most common cause of infection is hair penetrating the skin. For this reason, it is very important not to let hair enter the skin. As long as thorough preoperative sterilization procedures are adhered to, it is rare for infection to develop (Figure 8–10).

In cases of infection, the patient should be started on antibiotics and anti-inflammatory medication, and the thread should be removed if there is no response to treatment after one week.

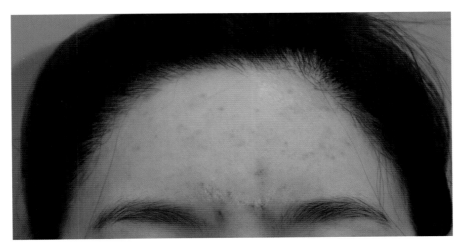

Figure 8–10. Inflammatory response after monofilament thread insertion in the glabella

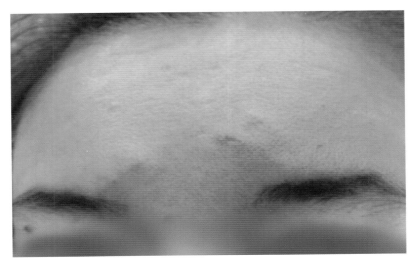

Figure 8–11. Inflammatory response after forehead and glabella thread lifting

SECTION 9

Nerve Injury

Although nerve injury can occur rarely after thread lifting, the procedure is performed carefully to minimize tissue damage and avoid areas with a high density of nerves. If possible, using cannulas rather than needles can reduce the risk of nerve injury.

Patients often have difficulty closing their eyes or downturned oral commissures after surgery, but this is usually a transient phenomenon caused by the anesthesia, and symptoms disappear after one day.

SECTION 10

Scarring

Because thread lifting is generally performed with a thin needle, scarring is not usually an issue. However, needle marks can last longer than expected in certain susceptible or keloid-prone patients; these tendencies should be checked in advance.

Rarely, hair loss can occur at the surgical site. We think that this is probably due to the thread being inserted in the surface layer, causing damage to the hair follicles. Therefore, when inserting the thread in the scalp area, it is important for the surgeon to place the thread in a deeper layer.

SECTION 11

Parotid Gland Injury

In rare cases, adverse effects can be caused by parotid gland injury. If postoperative pain and swelling is observed in the region of the parotid gland, parotid gland injury should be suspected. Since parotid gland injury can lead to further adverse effects (e.g., skin fistula), this should be treated aggressively with strong broad-spectrum antibiotics (Table 8–1).

In order to avoid these adverse effects, when placing the cannula for thread insertion, the surgeon should pinch the skin and be careful not to place the cannula too deep.

Table 8–1. Parotid gland injury

1) Compressionn
2) serial aspiration
3) Medical treatment Preventive antibiotic treatment: 5–7 days Augmentin 500 mg, 3 times/day Doxycycline 100 mg, 2 times/day (for patients with penicillin allergy)
4) Botulinum toxin A: also used for its anticholinergic effect

TEXTBOOK OF ABSORBABLE THREAD LIFTING

Index